HEALING SPORTS INJURIES

Healing Sports Injuries

A Hands-On Guide to Restorative Massage and Exercise

MARC CHASNOV AND STEVEN CLARK

Foreword by EAMONN COGHLAN

Photographs by MORT ENGEL

Illustrations by DANA BURNS

FAWCETT COLUMBINE • NEW YORK

A Fawcett Columbine Book
Published by Ballantine Books

Library of Congress Catalog Card Number: 86-92122

ISBN: 0-449-90271-4

Cover design by Tony Russo
Cover and text photographs by Mort Engel
Text design by Philip Wolf
Manufactured in the United States of America
First Edition: April 1988
10 9 8 7 6 5 4 3 2 1

To Alexander and Nicholas

CONTENTS

ACKNOWLEDGMENTS

Special thanks to Mel Berger from the William Morris Agency. Thanks to Eamonn Coghlan, Jerry Cahill, and Suzanne Kim for appearing in *Healing Sports Injuries*.

FOREWORD

I FIRST WENT TO SEE MARC CHASNOV three months before the 1984 Olympics. I was suffering from the recurrence of a stress fracture in my shinbone. To keep fit, I spent six hours a day riding a stationary bicycle and running in the deep end of a swimming pool. Although I knew I was probably fighting a losing battle in my determination to "strike gold" in Los Angeles, I was not ready to quit. What I needed most of all to get me through this time of crisis was someone who could really help me, understand my frustrations, and give me that extra bit of confidence to keep on trying.

I found that person in Marc Chasnov. His "magic" and expertise gave me what I had wanted and needed for years. His deep, penetrating massages were just what my aching body needed. He assured me that he could help me get the rest of my body into tip-top condition.

Ever since I began my running career at the age of twelve I had received regular massages from my physiotherapist in Ireland, Barney Crosby (now seventy-nine years old). In Europe, massage is considered one of the most important elements in training. However, when I came to the United States to attend Villanova University in 1972, I could not find anyone capable of giving a proper athletic, restorative, or rehabilitative massage. When I found Marc Chasnov, my twelve-year search ended.

Marc provides the perfect "remedy" for the athlete or nonathlete with his expert massage technique.

Regular massages leave my tight, aching muscles loose and relaxed and get rid of the lactic acid and N-bodies (as Marc calls them) that hinder my performance. I don't wait until I am injured or sore to receive massage, as massage also plays a major role in helping to prevent injuries. It is a regular part of my training program, and I consider it just as important as any track session.

Although my shinbone was not healed in time to allow me to compete in the 1984 Olympics, I was ready to begin a full exercise program created by Marc, not only to rehabilitate my weakened leg but also to help improve my athletic performance. I soon learned what "split squats," "power thrusts," and "box jumps" were, as drills like these gave me the extra power I needed without having to pound extra miles on the road. In fact, the program allowed me to reduce my weekly mileage from ninety-five to eighty miles, therefore decreasing the chance of reinjury. I can honestly say it was the result of this combined program of massage and exercise that enabled me to win eight out of eight indoor mile races during the 1985 season and to record the fastest indoor mile in the world that year.

Since I've met Marc, I've had no hesitation recommending him to my fellow sportsmen. Besides his knowledge and ability to get people better, he knows how to work with people. He has the gift of reassuring his patients and giving them the confidence they need during times of injury.

We all know that there is nothing worse than being told to just rest when you're injured. There is nothing better than experiencing the alternative—the Chasnov Method of healing, which says you can be cured sooner, better, and more completely than any other form of treatment. It worked for me, and I'm confident it can work for you, too.

EAMONN COGHLAN
*World Record Holder
for the Indoor Mile*

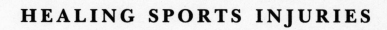

HEALING SPORTS INJURIES

INTRODUCTION

T HIS BOOK is dedicated to anyone whose body could feel better than it does right now.

We have all experienced our share of aches and pains. Going to specialists for treatment, many of us often end up feeling silly for having taken up their precious time. After all, the results of the X rays as well as the pop on our knee from that little hammerlike thing that tests our reflexes reveal that there's nothing to worry about. "Stay off it for a week," we're told. Or else we feel frustrated because we've just been condemned to a week of epsom salt baths, bed rest, and daily doses of codeine and Tylenol. And we're told to come back the following week to be X rayed and to discuss other treatments—such as surgery or an end to all physical activity—if there is no improvement.

Yet, there is a better way!

We can begin by taking a hard look at where our ideas on good health have come from and how they have changed in a world of high-tech exercise equipment and the existence of every kind of health specialist under the sun. This book will help you understand why you think the way you do about what's good (or what you think is good) for your body. By learning my philosophy, which I call the Chasnov Method, you will gain a more progressive and updated view of what a healthy body actually is and, most important, learn how to help yourself and others get better and stronger.

All it takes is a willingness to learn, to be self-critical, and to be dedicated to creating a better you!

The Chasnov Method is personal. It reaches out to all of us—from those who have experienced frustration with an injury to those who need to know how to design a training program that will make them stronger. The Chasnov Method, in fact, isn't totally new; its principles have been around in one form or another for centuries.

So, as modern, intelligent people of the 1980s, how have we been influenced and molded into our present impressions of health?

To start with, we have become a society dependent on machines. With more of the hard and demanding labor being performed by machines, fewer physical demands are being placed on the body. The same holds true for the mind, with computers doing much of our laborious thinking for us.

On the other side of the coin, more leisure time allows us energy for other interests, such as sports and recreation. Some people may be more interested in their jobs, while others prefer to concentrate on their leisure time. Regardless, everyone wants to do what he or she likes without worrying if he or she can physically or mentally accomplish it.

The public's attitude toward health is changing as well. Fifty years ago you probably would have been told that the injury to your back or your shoulder was due to rheumatism or lumbago. This would not have surprised you, because your father and grandfather had it too. Every time you had this pain, it was a case of "your rheumatism acting up," and you would get out the mustard plaster and apply it to the affected area. In those days, if you had such a problem, you talked to your family and friends, satisfied that with their advice you would be able to take care of yourself without needing to rush off to a health practitioner.

Traditions were handed down from generation to generation in each family. Only as a last resort would you seek trained medical advice. You had confidence in your family's treatment; after all, what was good enough for father or grandfather was good enough for you.

More recently, these "down-home" methods of treating ailments and injuries have given way to "professional advice." The family treatments of yesterday have become the old wives' tales of today. Nowadays, we trust specialists more than we trust ourselves. In this world of professionals, there are specialists for everything. One of the more recent specialties is "sports medicine." With more time for leisure, recreation, and sport, and with the advent of the fitness craze, more and more people are being injured. Realizing this, medical and nonmedical specialists in all fields are re-marketing themselves. Professionals who never before treated sports-related injuries are taking down their shingles and putting up new ones that read, "Sports Medicine." And they immediately triple their business without the need for any further training or knowledge. Non-sports-oriented people think to themselves that "if an athlete with an injury is going to a sports medicine specialist, and I am not nearly as proficient an athlete, then these experts definitely can help me."

The system has us at its mercy. There is too much choice, too much confusion, and too much public relations at the expense of too little personalized care. The natural good sense of the individual has suddenly taken a back seat to this professional advice. Yet, who should know your body better than you? Who can best care for it when it doesn't quite work properly? There must be a return to the individual, to the confidence that allows us to do what is right for our bodies. Only when we begin to believe in ourselves, when we realize that we have the ability to heal ourselves, will the balance of power return to the individual.

How Did the Chasnov Method Develop?

As a registered physical therapist, for years I was quite content teaching people to help themselves heal. Here

I was in my small office treating people hour after hour, usually twelve to sixteen hours a day, and giving them all sorts of exercises that were unknown to them. I was telling them things about their body that they never knew.

Continually, however, I was told by my patients, including one who would become my literary agent, that I had something to offer society. I know that what I do works, but how do you convey this to the public? After all, who was going to believe that most injuries to the body are soft-tissue injuries and that exercise and massage, the two oldest forms of treatment on record, will heal them? Taking this concept one step further, who was going to believe that a health professional who has a health license but not a medical degree can make people better?

I put these questions to rest when I looked back at my own medical history. Certain images flashed through my mind. First, the aloofness of the medical system when I was hurt; and then, my instinct to help myself through exercise and movement. This pattern of thought was reinforced by the number of people who came to see me for injuries that had been unsuccessfully treated by one, two, three, even four different medical professionals and who were restored to health with tissue-restorative massage and exercise.

I realized that in spite of how society presently observes current health practices, injured individuals really want to know what is wrong with them and how they can help themselves. This is when I decided to create a self-help guide dedicated to getting the body better.

My entire approach began developing in childhood. At age eight, I was told that I was sick with a "fever," which in fact was rheumatic fever. The strep infection that had left me partially deaf at age two had returned, this time to my heart. The year was 1959, a time when this condition offered limited choices for treatment: I ended up confined to a wheelchair. During this period, no one bothered to tell me that I could not bring my wheelchair outside the house, carry it down the steps and walk behind it, which I did if I felt good on a particular day.

I decided on my own to get up and become more active. Needless to say, I was surprised when I became weak, dizzy, and fatigued from walking just a few feet. Somehow, I decided to persevere. After all, only a month before I was climbing trees and getting into mischief like all the other kids.

I started by walking short distances. Finally, I made it around the block holding on to my wheelchair. Even though I was beginning to feel better, I always stayed near that wheelchair because I was "supposed" to be sick. After one year, when I was given a clean bill of health, I jumped out of my chair and ran outside to play. Even though I continued to take two penicillin pills each night for the next ten years, who cared? I was free.

This is the kind of initiative I shall be referring to as I discuss the need for individuals to assume an active role in their healing. At the age of ten, my right leg began to buckle and collapse during play. My knee swelled horribly, and from X rays, doctors diagnosed my condition as osteochondritis dissecans, a disease whose name I could not even pronounce.

I never remember anyone ever telling me exactly what my problem was. All I know is that a cast was put on my leg for ten months. During this time I ice-skated and played kickball, since no one told me I couldn't. I quickly became a kickball legend with my "extra powerful" leg. The day the cast came off, the doctor told me that I would have arthritis earlier than most people. I could not bend the knee. No therapy, no exercises were recommended—nothing but a handshake and a lollipop.

Again I went out to play. I jumped on my bicycle and started out by keeping my injured leg straight and pedaling with the left uninjured leg. After a few minutes, I told myself, "This does not feel right." The right pedal was all the way down when I put my right foot on it and thrust my left leg down. The right pedal came up forcing my right knee to bend. There was a tingling sensation and a ripping noise, followed by full bending motion in my knee.

Because of my own experiences with injuries and as a result of studying a book that my mother, a physical therapist, had used in school, I had become fascinated with muscles and movement at the age of thirteen. The book was about body movement (kinesiology). I began tracing the pictures and drawing the muscles and the other soft tissues. I did this over and over again. When I was tired of this book, I got others. I would study a muscle, see how it was attached to the body, and try to imagine where it was in my own body.

My father began teaching me weight lifting when I was seventeen, and I was excited because I wanted to become very strong. I learned the basics and I became stronger. One day I was doing a squat exercise, which involves a deep knee bend. Having progressed, during this time, from lifts of 100 pounds to nearly 300 pounds, I attempted to break this "300-pound barrier" but was having a problem. During one attempt, I squatted down and found I could not get up. I was alone, so there was no one to help me. When I threw my body back to rid myself of the weight, I miscalculated—the bar slid down my back and on the way down took the skin off my back and ribs. Two weeks later, however, still hurting, I made that 300-pound squat. Since then I have lifted more than 540 pounds in the same exercise. Not bad considering my childhood knee problems!

My interest in muscles and movement flourished in high school biology, and I decided that I wanted to study science in college.

At Cortland State University I experienced some disappointments. I had enrolled in a chemistry and biology course. To my dismay, biology consisted of studying plants and animals. Where was the human body? College biology majors, as I found out, never have to take anatomy, just physiology.

I ventured out on my own, walked into a book-store, and bought a book about massage. Since that time I have read every massage and exercise book I've been able to get my hands on.

From my studies at New York University's graduate program in physical therapy, my graduate degree from Columbia University Teacher's College in movement science, nearly two decades as a competitive weight lifter and private practice as a physical therapist in Westchester County, New York, I have developed an active yet conservative approach to getting the body better.

Perhaps the situation that influenced me most in my self-education occurred after I graduated from physical therapy school. During a weight lifting competition, I hurt my shoulder and elbow. After X rays, I was told that my right elbow and shoulder were both dislocated. The specialist put the joints back in place, put my arm in a sling, and told me I would not be able to lift again. Imagine, my entire future determined on the spot!

I decided to heal myself. At this time I was supervising a physical therapy department, and I asked my staff members to massage my elbow and shoulder. I used ultrasound to reduce pain and electrical muscle stimulation to strengthen the muscle while I began to force it through the gentlest of motions. After seven months of my own therapeutic program I was barely able to lift a forty-five-pound bar without pain. But later, after staying in the program, I won the New York State Weight Lifting Championships and placed in the top five in the American Weight Lifting Championships.

No one has ever given me a list of dos and don'ts. Whenever I was sick or injured, I just had a natural inclination to want to know more. I decided early on that since I was not given much solid advice about improving the well-being of the body, I would take it upon *myself* to get better. I learned, after sustaining a variety of injuries and gaining experience as a competitive weightlifter, that movement made me feel better, although at times it was difficult and extremely painful. I have since become convinced that mobility through exercise along with massage greatly accelerates the healing process.

These ideas form the basis of the Chasnov Method of getting the body better. The method approaches the body from a more complete point of view—that the body is one unit, not a collection of isolated parts. When one part is out of sync, the whole unit is affected. To understand how the body works best as a total entity, we need to look at the most important area of the body: its foundation.

Section One

Building the Foundation

IN ORDER TO HELP YOU understand the body better, we must take a more serious look at how it is made, the actual composition of the musculoskeletal system. The approach I take here may appear somewhat technical, but on the whole the ideas are easy to understand. These concepts are crucial to our comprehension of what makes up a healthy body and how to speed up the healing process when it's not so healthy.

In the early stages of our fetal development, the body develops in three layers: inner (endoderm), middle (mesoderm) and outer (ectoderm). The middle layer, the mesoderm, gives rise to a substance called *mesenchyme*. It is mesenchyme that provides the source of all connective tissue, both hard and soft, in our bodies. All the muscles and bones—that is, the entire framework of the human organism—are composed of hard and soft tissue.

We all know that every structure in the universe has some point or area within it from which it gets its strength. Flowers and trees are supported by their roots. All man-made structures—from single-story homes to skyscrapers—are supported by their foundations.

Similarly, the human body gets its strength and framework from a center point. However, unlike its stationary, rooted counterparts, the body needs to experience movement in order to function and survive. After all, it is through movement that we perform all of the basic functions of day-to-day life. We express feel-

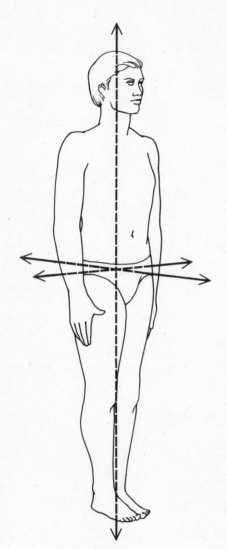

ings, demonstrate our abilities and creations, and respond to our environment with our bodies. Therefore, in order for the body to operate with maximum efficiency, our movement must come from a strong and stable base. A solid foundation is essential for us to be able to increase ease of movement, prevent injuries in daily life, and develop higher levels of performance.

Using a theoretical model, this center of gravity in the body is located by:

1. Looking at the body from the front or back and dividing it from head to foot into right and left sides.

2. Looking at it from the same viewpoint and dividing it according to body weight into equal upper and lower halves.

3. Looking at the body from the side and dividing it into front and back halves.

The point at which all three lines meet is the body's center of gravity. The area that surrounds this center is the *core*. The core, or midsection, is made up of all body tissues, but we are concentrating on muscles and bones. Remember that this is a theoretical construct designed to help us better visualize the development of the body and to prepare for exercise training to strengthen the core. In later chapters the core should simply be considered the focus of the body's foundation. All movement, no matter how minimal or exerting, comes from the core.

The Skeletal System

If you can read this book, you are old enough to have seen a full human skeleton in a museum, a biology class, or as the high point of a horror movie. Thus, our associations with skeletons are simultaneously full of fascination and horror. But regardless of what you think of it, the fact is that the human skeleton serves its purpose extremely well, that of forming a framework for the body. A tribute to its structure, after all, is its durability—skeletons can survive for millennia.

There are over two hundred bones that make up the skeleton. These bones are connected in a way that allows us to stand upright in the most efficient manner possible. As a result of the great stresses and demands placed upon the bones throughout one's lifetime, each portion of every bone fits together to support movement. For example, the pelvis is flat and bowllike to support the upper body. The roundness of the top of the thighbone permits movement. Every time we take a running step or bend over to pick something up, hundreds of these "connections" work simultaneously.

The functions of the bones are to:
- Provide the hard framework of the body
- Protect the inner organs
- Provide the crucial points for muscles to attach so that movement can take place
- Participate in the production of red blood cells

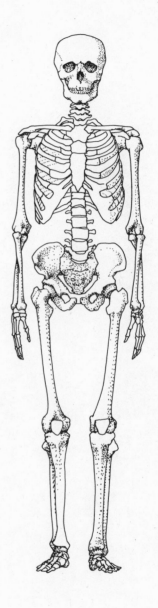

The Joints

The location where two bones meet is a joint. The joint is supported by the shape of the bones that form it, the cartilage at the ends or between the bones, the ligaments that hold bones together, and the surrounding muscles. Joints involved in multiple movements have a closed capsule that contains fluid for lubricating the joints.

The major joints of the body are:
- Shoulders, elbows, wrists, fingers (upper body)
- Spinal column, sacroiliac (trunk)
- Hips, knees, ankles, feet (lower body)

The smooth functioning of all joints is crucial to

healthy movement, but for our immediate purposes, we want to focus on the core joints, specifically the pelvis and the spinal column.

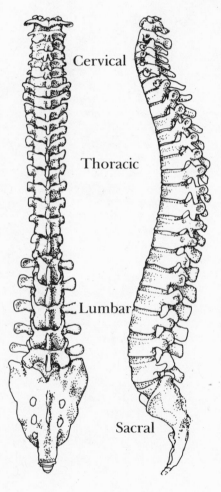

Cervical

Thoracic

Lumbar

Sacral

The Pelvis

The very shape and location of the pelvis reveal its role. Situated in the middle of the skeleton, the pelvis actually surrounds the theoretical center of the body. For this reason, the pelvis is the primary foundation bone of the skeleton.

Its shape—broad, flaring, and bowllike—allows the pelvis to support the weight of the entire upper body and distributes this weight to the lower body. The pelvis also absorbs shock from the lower body. The pelvis area alone has more muscles than any other area of the body. Many muscles begin, end, or cross over here.

The Spinal Column

If observed from the front or back, the spine normally appears straight. When viewed from the side, however, it looks like a stretched-out reversed letter S. Nature has given us these curves so that the body can absorb shock and large amounts of energy.

Four of these curves exist in the adult spine. Curves 1 and 3 are arched forward. These are, respectively, the neck (cervical) and the lower back (lumbar) curves. Curves 2 and 4 are rounded backward and retain the curves that are present from birth. These are, respectively, the middle back (thoracic) and the tailbone (sacral) curves.

We are born with a big, rounded spine. As infants, when we look up while lying on our stomachs, the neck arch curve develops. This curve permits us, as children, to observe the world with our eyes looking straight ahead. By the time we are one year old, we begin to stand and walk, and the arch of the lower back develops to absorb the weight of the upper body. The arches in the sacral and thoracic area, however, remain rounded throughout our lives.

The thoracic and sacral curves are attached to other bones, the ribs and the pelvis; these attachments give the spine more support and stability. The neck and back curves, meanwhile, do not have any extra bone support (that is, no rib attachments). Consequently, we have more freedom of movement in these areas. By the same token, the lack of added stability in these areas makes them very susceptible to common soft-tissue injuries.

The four curves in the spine (two arched backward, two forward) counterbalance each other in reducing vertical pressure on the vertebral column as a whole. This balancing act gives rise to the functions of the spinal column, which are:

- To support and transfer weight from the head, arms, and shoulders to the lower body
- To absorb shock from the upper body and protect the spinal cord and nerves
- To connect the lower body at the pelvic/ sacroiliac joint

The Soft-Tissue System

All tissue in the body, with the exception of bone and cartilage, is soft tissue. A high percentage of injuries, as we will see, involve the soft-tissue system. Areas with great mobility (neck, back, hip, shoulder, knee) have more soft tissue in relation to hard tissue. The muscular system is composed of the largest percentage of soft tissue in the body.

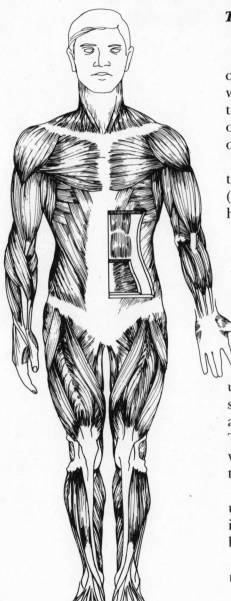

The Muscles

There are over six hundred muscles in the body, constituting 40 percent or more of our total body weight. Muscles come in all shapes and sizes according to their function. The majority of them run lengthwise or vertically; some have a crosswise orientation. Still others are a combination of the two.

Generally, muscles that run lengthwise along the body are associated with motion, while the others (horizontal) tend to be used for support. All muscles have the following functions:

- Contractibility—the ability to contract or shorten and, as they contract, to develop tension
- Extensibility—the capacity to stretch
- Irritability—the ability to respond to stimuli from the nervous system
- Elasticity—the ability to return to their original size and length after being stretched

Basically speaking, muscles shorten or contract upon receiving a signal from the nervous system. If the signal is deliberate or voluntary, the muscle shortens and pulls its two connecting "points" closer together. The signal may also be reflexive or involuntary. This is where the nervous system instructs the muscles to stop their motions or limit them for protection from injury.

Muscles are also involved in holding the body upright against gravity. This low level of muscle activity allows the muscles to help the joints support the body's weight without straining and becoming injured.

For our purposes, the remaining soft tissue in the body consists of the following:

- Ligaments—strong tissue that connects bone to bone
- Tendons—narrow bands or rounded cords that attach muscles to bone
- Fascia—sheets of connective tissue that enclose and support muscles

- Aponeuroses—broad, flat sheets of tendon
- Retinaculam—a small, localized type of tissue that holds the tendons in place
- Bursae—saclike cavities between the muscles, tendons, and bones that reduce friction
- Joint capsules—two-layered structures: the outer layer for support and the inner layer for lubrication

Order of Control of the Body

Although we have not yet discussed the nervous system, it is the function of this system to direct control over the body.

Movement:

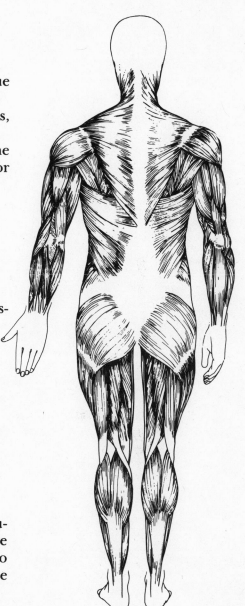

Nervous System
controls
Muscular System
controls
Bone System

It is important to realize that this order influences exercise prescription and rehabilitation. One cannot treat just a bone or a joint. One always has to teach the brain to direct the muscles to control the bone as a total coordinated process.

Chapter 1
POSTURE

HOW MANY TIMES have you heard someone say, "Stand up straight," "sit back," "stop slouching," "pull your stomach in," "push your chest out," "pull your shoulders back?"

We usually respond instantaneously to these commands, changing our position to what we interpret as "correct posture." The problem? Less than a minute or two later, when attention is no longer focused on our posture, we revert back to our natural position, usually a slight slouch of some sort. What is important is that we become conditioned to being aware of better posture, even though we may have no idea physiologically of exactly what posture is.

If you ask ten people, "What is posture?" they may all be able to tell you what makes it bad, but it is unlikely that anyone will know what makes it good. Female gymnasts are supposed to have good posture, yet many have extreme forward arches in the lower back. Dancers are considered to have good posture, yet they always walk with their legs and feet turned out. Military people standing at attention are regarded as good postural specimens; however, their posture is so static and straight that it is unnatural. The fact of the matter is that no one at any age has perfect posture and that the term *good posture* may be only good on paper.

Posture is defined as the relationship of your body to itself and of your body to space. In order for posture to be good and efficient, it must "work" at both levels. The female gymnast, for instance, meets the

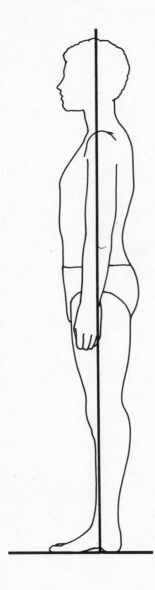

second qualification—good posture in space—but because of the extreme arch in the lower back she lacks good posture relative to her own body.

Although reference to posture can be made in any position, historically the posture of the human body has usually been discussed in the upright position.

Looking at an imaginary line drawn down the middle of the body from a side view, we should ideally see it pass through the center of the ear, the center of the shoulder, the head of the thighbone, and the middle of the ankles.

Postural Changes

As infants and children our spines are not fully matured, but our postural habits are beginning to develop. These habits will condition how our bodies move as we grow older. By the age of ten, all the mature curves in the spine and the basic pattern of body alignment in the upright position are fully developed.

In childhood, proper postural habits must be learned or the bones and joints will not attain their proper alignment as they mature. During adolescence, as the body undergoes its growth spurts and acquires secondary sex characteristics, any bad habits from childhood will be intensified.

Unless we are extremely disciplined in our late teens or early twenties, we no longer have time or organized instruction for exercise. Any injury sustained while working, running, doing an exercise improperly, or falling causes a change in our posture.

At forty years of age, as we settle down in our careers and become more sedentary, we have a tendency to gain weight, lose muscle tone, and experience further deterioration in our posture.

By sixty years of age, years of neglect, tight imbalanced muscles, and poor exercise habits cause pain and loss of function. We may have to fight so hard to stand upright or hold our head up that the majority of our body's energy is used simply fighting gravity. As a result, we tire easily. We tend to be always stiff and achy and we may find ourselves thinking that things are not as easy today as they were yesterday.

Too often we accept this postural "decay" as being part of the natural course of our lives. Society dictates this to us. We are born helpless, we get stronger, we struggle through middle age and get older, and, we are told, there is nothing we can do to change it. What people do not realize is that good postural habits can be developed during childhood, adolescence, and early adulthood; this prevents problems thirty, forty, fifty years down the road. Your present postural alignment, regardless of your age, can be changed for the better by following a structured program of exercise and massage as laid out in this book. Whether you are fifteen or seventy-five, working on maintaining and improving your posture is something you should commit to for the rest of your life.

Common features of poor posture are the following:

1. Forward head, relative to the line of gravity
2. Rounded, sloped shoulders
3. Rounded upper, middle back
4. Arched lower back
5. Anterior-tilted pelvis
6. Hyperextended knees
7. Flat feet

Posture is not only important with respect to movement, it affects other systems as well. A tight, rounded upper body and shoulders, for example, will prevent the lungs from filling completely, reducing breathing capacity.

Another, more recently recognized problem I have seen relating to poor posture is temporomandibular joint disease (TMJ). Presently, I am treating a number of people suffering from this condition who

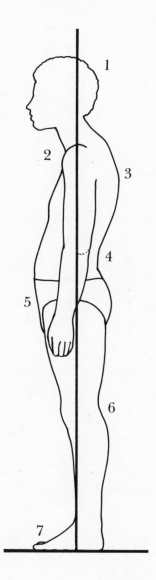

have been sent to me by dentists. As a result of poor alignment of their head, jaw, and neck in relation to their upper body, these people experience difficulty and pain when chewing. This imbalance also triggers headaches, neck pain, and dizziness.

Bad posture can also cause you to tilt your head downward, making your eyes compensate by looking up in order to see. This in turn causes an increased forward arch in the neck. These competing forces, as we may expect, cause neck pain. Rounding the shoulders and upper back puts greater pressure on the vertebrae and the discs between them. Disc degeneration and arthritis may occur if this process is left uncorrected.

It must be stressed, as it is over and over in this book, that the body works as a unit. A weak link in one area will be overcompensated for or absorbed in another. In the case of rounded shoulders, for example, the body automatically finds a new center point, a new "point of gravity," to compensate for the forward, slumped shoulders. The bad part is that this new set point may pull the head forward or increase the forward arch in the lower back.

What we must realize is that bad posture is not limited to the nonactive. Athletes who are well accomplished in their fields are not exempt from feeling the effects of poor posture. Take the case histories of two of my former patients. Bruce works in a health center and is a skilled enough distance runner to have won a major East Coast marathon, a run of 26.2 miles, in under two hours and twenty minutes. This is especially remarkable considering Bruce's posture. When he first came to me, his shoulders were terribly rounded and his upper back was drastically sloped. Yet, throughout his career as a high school and college athlete and as a student of physical education no one—neither a coach, trainer, nor physician—ever questioned his posture. They just figured that if he could run that well, he must not have much of a problem.

Like many other people's, Bruce's poor posture

over the years had resulted in a forward thrust of the neck and head, rounded shoulders, rounded upper back, and arched lower back. Because the postural alignment of the skeleton is disturbed, the muscles have constantly to work harder to maintain normal alignment. The muscles tighten in an effort to prevent future postural shifts (although these will actually continue to occur). The body appears to limit its own motion in order to secure its upright position. So much energy is utilized for posture that nothing is left over for other skills. The tightened muscles also fatigue more easily due to a decrease in local blood circulation in the muscle. In fact, a negative cycle follows in which the metabolism and health of the muscle are disturbed.

So, it was no wonder that Bruce was fatiguing so easily. In running, a rounded back does not permit the upper body to move properly. This negates any benefits of a good arm swing and limits proper rotation of the upper body. If your upper body does not work efficiently, neither will your lower body. Bruce's breathing suffered as well. The tightness in his chest muscles prevented his lungs from filling to capacity. This reduced both the amount of air getting to his lungs and the oxygen in the blood going to his muscles. Without an abundant supply of oxygen in his blood, Bruce not only tired easily but was more susceptible to injury. It was amazing to examine the internal chain of events that could take place just because of bad posture. What a mess for an active person in his twenties!

Bruce began seeing me when he started to have pain in his back from extremely spasmed muscles. Upon examining him, I began treating him with massage and prescribed a series of specific, corrective exercises that would gradually increase in difficulty. I told him that by following this program, he would eventually run the same time—and hopefully better—without expending as much energy.

The purpose of massage is to restore the health of the muscle, which will then reduce tightness. Exercises are prescribed in conjunction with massage to stretch the tightened area and tighten the stretched areas. I recommended stretching exercises for Bruce's tight neck and lower back muscles and tightening exercises for his upper back. This positive-reinforcement program of massage and exercise was so effective that Bruce was running more efficiently and pain-free within months—and he was looking much better, too.

Better posture can affect other, nonathletic areas, such as voice quality, for example. Alexis, another patient, is an opera singer. She herself believed, and correctly so, that better posture would improve her performance. I treated her for neck and upper-back-muscle tightness and gave her exercises to improve her posture. The treatment released the tension in her head, neck, and vocal apparatus, which had been compromised by poor posture. Not only did her posture improve after treatment, but she reported a great improvement in her singing.

A Developmental View

Shortly after birth, a baby's *in utero* rounded position remains, but diminishes slightly as the neuromuscular system matures. The rounded position slowly relaxes and the body "unfolds." At this time, when the child is two or three months old, the *extensors* (muscles involved when we "open" as opposed to when we flex our bodies, as in curling up) become more active. The infant begins to use his extensors by lying on his stomach and lifting up his head.

The infant quickly advances to a position where he arches his upper and lower body while lying on his stomach. Soon, he progresses to leaning on his hands and knees, kneeling, half kneeling and half standing, and then fully standing. He begins to use his arms and legs for balance and coordination. This is where he begins kicking with his legs while moving his arms simultaneously, a precursor to walking. Already, within the first year of life, posture begins to develop.

Posture and Evolution

My major hypothesis on posture revolves around the ratio of time for the developmental process of our ancestors and modern man versus life expectancy then and now. Prehistoric man's life expectancy was barely thirty to forty years. As we approach the twenty-first century, we are living an average of two to three times longer than our ancestors. We can only guess that prehistoric children progressed through the same developmental stages we do now within the same time period (12 to 18 months). However, now that we currently live three times longer, perhaps this development may not be sufficient to sustain our posture for all our lives (witness all the aches, pains, and injuries associated with the aging process). This means that we have to do more to reinforce normal development, not only in infancy and childhood, but throughout our entire lives.

Conscious versus Subconscious

Historically, experts on posture and body movement have had a running battle over how posture can be altered or if it can be changed at all. Generations of mothers have verbally encouraged their children to develop good posture habits. Only twenty or so years ago, it was not uncommon for young girls to spend the better part of their evenings walking around the house with schoolbooks on their heads, convinced by their mothers or teachers that this would give them better posture and make them more desirable.

So we could all take a few minutes each day to stroll around the house with a best-seller on our heads! Unfortunately, again, the results are only temporary—what we need to realize is that it takes a lot of hard work to make good posture a way of life.

Certain exercise techniques suggest that posture can be improved by using visual cues to teach your body good habits. For example, if you envision yourself walking with a balloon and string attached to your head, your neck will elongate and so will your body, resulting in a more upright posture.

Visualization exercises are most important and should be practiced, but this is only the beginning of the process. By exercising properly, you automatically hold your head up because you are stronger. By doing exercises repetitively and continuously, your muscles subconsciously learn to function in a better position for longer periods of time.

Later in this book you will be introduced to exercises that will strengthen and improve your body by correcting postural deficiencies and repairing and preventing injuries. However, there are several basic stretching exercises that will stretch out those tight areas associated with bad posture. By doing these exercises regularly, you should begin to see and feel improvement. These exercises, however, are simply intended to prepare you for the more strenuous strengthening exercises later in the book. They will not significantly strengthen or improve range of motion by themselves.

Stretching Exercises

1. *Neck Tilt.* Tight muscles in your head and neck may result in the head being arched forward. The idea here is both to stretch out the muscles in the back of the neck and to tighten the muscles in the front. As a result, the spine becomes better aligned and the muscles that once forced the neck into bad posture now reduce the curvature of the neck.

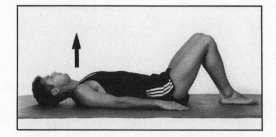 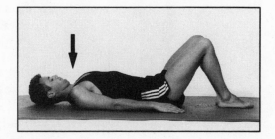

<u>Steps:</u> Lie on your back with your hands at your side, your legs bent, and your feet on the floor. Bend your head so as to bring the chin down toward your chest. Hold this position for two seconds and slowly release out of it. If you can touch the back of your neck to the ground, your neck-head alignment approaches a more correct position.

2. *Pelvic Tilt.* The lower back often has problems similar to those in the neck. If done repeatedly, the pelvic tilt will help stretch out the lower back.

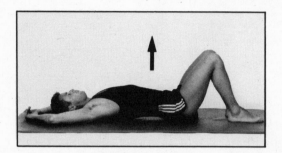
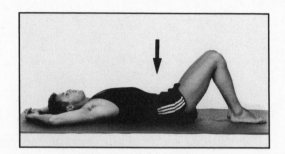

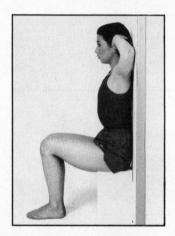

Steps: Lie on your back on the floor with your feet flat and your knees bent. Tighten and pull your abdominal muscles in and squeeze your buttocks together without lifting it off the ground. The pelvis will tilt slightly up while you press the lower part of your back flat on the floor. Again hold for two seconds and release slowly.

3. *Chestaways.* This exercise will work on the over-roundedness of the middle-back area. The chestaway will help stretch out the muscles in the upper back. It is probably the most difficult of the stretching exercises.

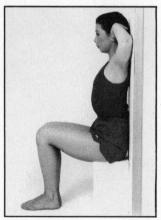

Steps: Move into this exercise gradually. Sit on a bench, with feet flat on the floor so that ankles, knees, and hips are at 90-degree angles. Hold the abdominal area firm and place the lower back flat against the wall. The lower and upper back and the back of the head should touch the wall. Eyes should be directed straight ahead. Hold arms at the sides of body against the wall.

   If your lower back cannot touch the wall, elevate your feet by placing them on a book. Practice moving into this position and holding it for two seconds before releasing.

   Once this portion of the exercise has been mastered, clasp your hands behind your head and press the backs of your elbows into the wall. Hold this for two seconds and release.

The most advanced stage of this exercise is to hold the original position when your hands are clasped behind your head and the elbows are pressed into the wall. Move your chest away from the wall without moving any other part of your body.

4. Hanging Exercises. This exercise is for stretching out the upper and lower back and the neck.

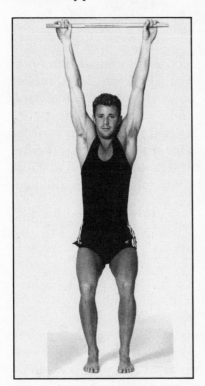 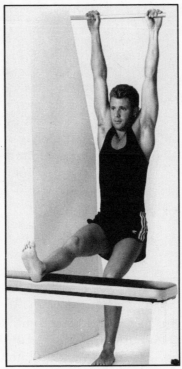 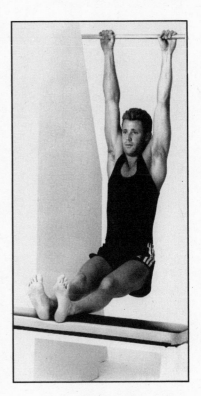

<u>Steps:</u> Place a bar in a doorway. Hold the bar with the palms of your hands facing away from you. In a standing position, squat down. In a sitting position form an L, with one and then both legs 90 degrees to the trunk of your body.

5. All-Fours to Side Sitting. This exercise will work the tight muscles in the lower back.

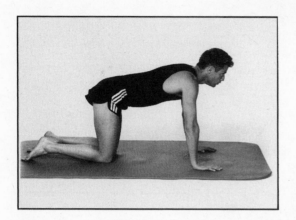 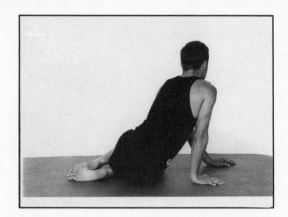

Steps: On the floor, place yourself in an all-fours position (on your hands and knees). Slowly swing the left side of your pelvis down toward your left hand. Hold this position for two seconds. Return to the starting position. If you can touch your left pelvis to your left wrist (or right pelvis to right wrist), your lateral trunk muscles, shoulder, and pelvic mobility are good. These exercises are also good for stretching the middle and lower back.

6. Twists.

Steps: Sitting straight, keep your feet together. Extend your arms straight to the side at shoulder level while holding a stick. Rotate your arms and your body to the left as far as possible, turning your head to look over your left shoulder. Keep your knees together and feet flat. Repeat, rotating your body to the right. You are within normal limits if you can rotate your body with the stick close to a 90-degree angle. You should work toward this slowly.

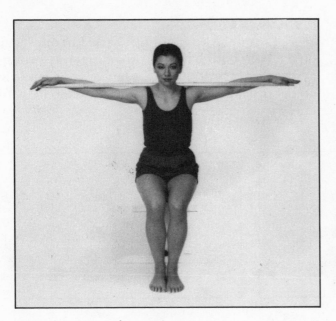 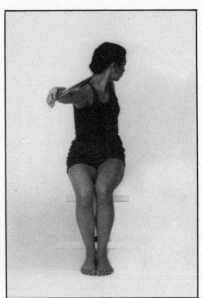

7. Trunk Rotation, Side Lying.

Steps: Lie on the floor on your side, with your top leg bent at a 90-degree angle. Keeping the knee in place, twist your upper body so that both shoulders touch the floor. Repeat on the other side.

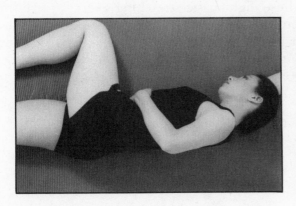 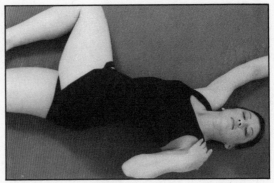

8. Knees to Chest.

Steps: Lie on the floor on your back. Lift one leg up and hold it with both hands. Bring it in toward your chest, moving your head up as if to meet your knee. Repeat on the other side. Now do the same exercise with both knees to your chest.

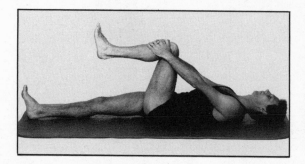
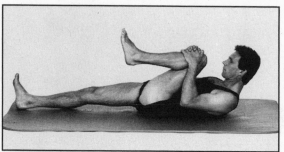
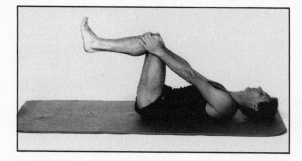
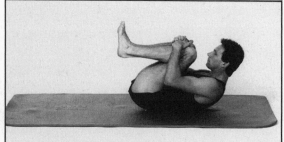

These eight basic stretching exercises will improve your posture, loosen your muscles, and prepare them for more demanding exercises. Later, and most importantly, you will learn to strengthen them so that they become less prone to injury and more resistant to pain.

Sports

W E ALL ENJOY PARTICIPATING IN SPORTS, whether
it means competing in our regular Wednesday-night
squash game or running sixty to eighty miles a week.
Better posture may mean being able to perform the
same activity with less strain, giving you the stamina to
do much more. An example of this would be Bruce, the
marathoner. By making his posture and movement
better, he has the potential to improve in his specialty.

The athlete with poor posture has an added dis-
advantage in that participating in a sports activity not
only reinforces the bad habit but puts the body under
greater strain and makes it more prone to injury. In
any movement, the motion itself is the product of all its
participating segments. If the movement is not accomplished in a coordinated way, there is a greater chance
of injury. Bill is a patient of mine who has such poor
upper-torso posture that every time he plays squash,
he has restricted use of his arm. The result: a case of
severe tennis elbow.

Bill came to see me complaining of pain in his
right elbow. He had been told he had tennis elbow, and
when I first examined him, he could not straighten his
arm because his elbow was fixed in a bent position. He
also did not have full movement in his shoulders and
back because of the muscle tightness. It was obvious to
me that Bill had an exaggerated forward arch in his
lower back. When asked to twist his body from right to
left, he could not do it.

Since he plays a sport that involves extensive
twisting and he cannot turn his entire body properly,
he ends up playing more of an arm or wrist-shoulder
game than a total-body game. By not straightening his
arm completely, the muscles in the front and back of
his elbow have contracted to such a degree that he has a
permanent bend in his elbow. It is clear that a weakness
in one part has resulted in problems in other parts of
his body. Each linkage has broken down in some man-

ner. The lower back has tightened, then the shoulder blade, then the shoulder, the elbow, and the forearm. At any one time, either or all of these areas could cause him physical discomfort or injury.

In order for him to play and feel better, he has to develop more body rotation. This means that he has to have more flexibility in his lower and upper back and that the muscles in his shoulder blades have to control the shoulder area so that he begins to use his arm, elbow, and wrist better.

I never expected Bill to stop playing squash. Yet he will have to spend much more time performing the rehabilitative exercises than actually playing in order to counteract the poor body mechanics he has acquired through poor movement habits. The best chance he has of not injuring himself further is to limit playing time for the four to six months it will take for him to improve his arm tightness and his overall posture. When he returns to his game, he will be able to use the parts of his body more fully and efficiently. The components of the movement will be more effective, and he will have a better sum of all his participating parts.

A woman came to see me complaining of problems with her shoulder from playing tennis. One specialist had diagnosed her injury as a shoulder dislocation when in fact she had an irritation of her shoulder tendons. Although her sore shoulder had a little more motion than the other, no one had considered an important part of her medical history: She had had a surgical procedure in which some of the muscle in the chest area had been removed.

This surgery and the lack of postoperative rehabilitation threw off the natural posture and balance of her shoulder musculature. As a result of this surgery, she was now using the tendons and ligaments of the shoulder more than her muscles. The exercises I gave her reinforced her shoulder and strengthened the area. When she returned to playing tennis, her shoulder was healed and she did not have to worry about reinjuring that part of her body any longer.

Many of us live the life of the "weekend warrior." Used to sitting at our desks most of the week, we try to make up for lost time on the weekends by jogging or bicycling or playing touch football, tennis, or basketball. Or we run to fitness centers to receive the benefits of aerobics or weight machines. A ball of fire on the weekends fizzles out by Monday, and too much too soon leaves us with injuries.

We find we have problems staying still for too long, whether it be while driving a bus or sitting at a word processor. The result of this inactivity is sore, stiff muscles and joints. There are a number of very basic things you can do to break up the monotony of working for hours in one place doing the same task. For starters, look into buying a chair that affords you better support. Sit with your hips and knees at 90-degree angles instead of sitting slumped over or to one side. Take frequent breaks to prevent the buildup of postural tension. Try to take an exercise break for five minutes every hour you work, at least standing up and sitting back down several times and shrugging your shoulders. We can reduce pain and feel better about ourselves by improving our posture. It helps to know how one's body is held together. In the next section, you will be able to put the major components of the Chasnov Method together for the purpose of making the body better through healing, prevention, and correction.

Section Two

Restorative Therapy

MY HANDS AND FINGERS are the tools of my trade. I use these tools to dig for the root of a problem and probe for answers. As my patients can attest, I literally probe and dig! What my eyes cannot see, my fingertips feel. And for you to understand what my touch tells me and how I use this information to help you, we need to examine how the body reacts to stress and inflammation. The roots of my expertise are knowing the body's way of "getting irritated" when upset and how it "regains its composure."

My lectures to high school and college health classes and to fitness groups concerning tissue-restorative therapy begin on the most basic of levels: If you clean out the cobwebs from your grade-school studies of science, you will recall the smallest complete structure of living form in the universe that can function on its own as a unit is a cell.

Amazing things go on within the cells of our body. It is here that chemical reactions occur. All energy comes from and is released from here. Life develops here—all within a microscopic cell or a group of cells!

Since groupings of similar cells make up the tissues, they play an important role in keeping the tissue healthy. Cellular continuity is the basis for our understanding of what happens when something goes wrong with the body.

As discussed in section 1, "Building the Foundation," the major musculoskeletal tissues of the body are the bones and joints, while the major soft tissues are

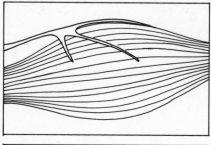

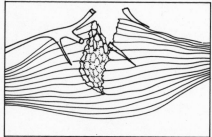

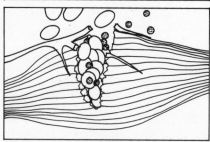

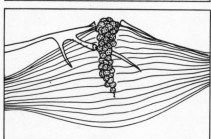

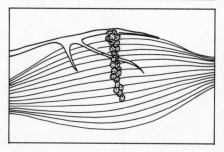

muscles, tendons, ligaments, bursae, fascia, retinacula and aponeuroses. Communication between cells is crucial in keeping these tissues healthy. Technically, this means there must be a smooth exchange of important fluids and nutrients both within and between the cells.

Tissue injury occurs when this network of cells has been disturbed. There is an interruption of continuity in the tissue and the body reacts naturally to stop it. The main indications of an inflammation are swelling, redness, heat, and pain in the affected area.

Inflammation may last anywhere from twenty-four to ninety-six hours, or even longer depending on the seriousness of the injury. It is therefore very important for us to take an active role in the healing process as soon as possible after the initial injury (once it has been determined that there is no injury to the bone). I practice active therapy to rid the injured areas of excess inflammation as quickly and as completely as possible, and I do this by creating a comprehensive program of massage and exercise. These two forms of treatment are further discussed in chapter 5, "Healing."

The normal healing mechanism after every soft-tissue injury, big or small, is the attempt to correct what is wrong. As a result of a tear in the soft tissue, post-inflammatory waste products build up. Eventually, the buildup of these waste products becomes so great that the original purpose of the inflammation, healing, is counteracted. The buildup of "debris" in the tissue must be diminished to allow for normal body processes to occur.

Regular restorative tissue massage in conjunction with active exercises will "cleanse" the tissues of these excess waste products. Although massage and exercise are themselves inflammatory to a small degree, this inflammation is necessary to encourage the healing process. Used together, massage and exercise are the best and most natural forms of healing.

Experience has shown me again and again that massage and exercise work better in healing soft-tissue injuries than any other methods including rest and inactivity. Unless the injury involves a complete tear in the tissue or a broken bone, my methods can help!

The beginning of this section will explain how the body reacts to everyday wear and tear. It shows how muscles and other soft tissues are affected by muscle tears, strains, sprains, or muscle imbalances. You will understand why your muscles cramp or go into spasm and how these problems can be alleviated.

Better yet, you will learn how to become your own healer. You will be taught how to give hands-on treatment to family members and friends. You will be able to set up a "clinic" in your own home at little or no cost. And you will be given insights into those types of exercises that will strengthen the body and increase its range of motion for the purposes of repairing a tissue injury, preventing it from happening again, and raising the body to a higher level of performance.

Later chapters will focus on exercises that illustrate my philosophy of treating the patient as a whole person, not simply an injured muscle. We will also explore the most common passive forms of treating injuries, namely ice, heat, elevation, compression, and rest, and how to use them correctly to assist the healing process.

The Injury

You rise from your chair in what is usually a simple motion and suddenly, without warning, you find you cannot straighten up. You glance in the mirror and see yourself all bent over and unable to move. You're thinking, "Why am I in this predicament?" You actually don't care. All you want is for the pain to go away.

So what should you do? Do you stop moving or force your way up through the pain? Do you rub the sore area or leave it untouched? Should you take aspirin, go to bed, apply ice or heat to it? Who do you call for help?

In this type of situation, nothing else exists but the pain. The world around you is in limbo because all you can think about is your physical distress. And when you don't know what to do next, you panic!

Anyone who has ever lifted a heavy package, run for a bus, or sat behind a desk for any length of time has felt the discomfort of muscle pain. It may have been a dull ache that lasted a fleeting moment or discomfort so intense that it left you flat on your back for weeks.

Everyone responds differently to pain. Whether you have a high or low tolerance for pain, the one common denominator for all of us is if we're hurt, the pain must go. Quickly!

We use our muscles and soft tissues in everything we do. They are used vigorously to catch a ball, sing, or dance, less actively when we sit, read, or simply hold (unconsciously) our bodies upright against the force of gravity to allow us to stand erect.

Any motion is the result of many muscles working together. For any coordinated motion to occur, some muscles direct others, others oppose, and still others hold or fixate the area so that the motion can occur. Obviously, the more a muscle is used within normal ranges of motion, the better it works. If greater demands are placed on the muscle by using it for prolonged periods or in an unusual manner, it is more prone to becoming overused, imbalanced or injured.

In the case of a perfectly balanced body that works with the best possible coordination, the strain on the muscles is minimized. However, as is often the case, any slight deviation in posture or any extended overuse or underuse irritates the muscle. This kind of irritation can start with microtearing or bleeding in various areas of the muscle, a condition that may at first go unnoticed. Later, this can cause major swelling or spasm in the muscle, which we feel and usually cannot ignore.

The most common of basic muscle traumas is *myositis*, more commonly known as muscle soreness.

This problem usually plagues the weekend warrior, who works a forty-hour week and crams all his or her physical activity in on the weekends. On Saturday after tending the garden, defeating your neighbor in straight sets, and dancing at your sister-in-law's wedding, you feel like a million dollars. On Sunday, however, you can barely make it out of bed. Your muscles are suffering from their own version of a hangover.

Not all muscle problems, however, are a result of physical exertion. Since most of us spend our lives in a chronic state of nervous tension, our muscles are always being told to contract by our nervous system. This way they never get a chance to relax. By being in a constant state of tightness, they get used to that position.

Regardless of whether the muscles are overused, underused, or too tense, the body's natural way of protecting itself is the same.

Inflammation

When soft tissue is irritated, the process of inflammation immediately begins to heal the injured area. Blood rushes into the area to bombard the injury with nutrients. The swelling inside the cells causes them to leak fluid. The area becomes red, hard, and tight.

Without the normal blood supply and movement, the muscle fibers themselves, along with excess nutrients and dead blood cells, begin to come together and lump. I call these clumped areas of fibrotic tissue *nodular bodies* or N-bodies. I can feel these bumpy areas with my hands.

The N-bodies do not cause reactions themselves, but wreak havoc on the surrounding tissue. They take up space and put pressure on the nerves and blood vessels in healthy muscle tissue. The internal healing powers of the body are not sufficient to remove the N-bodies. This is the time when outside active sources of help are required.

Chapter 2

RESTORATIVE
MASSAGE

I GOT MY NICKNAME, MAGIC FINGERS, from a former associate, Joel Daunic, the athletic director at the college where I once worked, and one of the first to recognize my skills in treating injuries. Most people think that my reputation stems from my ability to do vigorous massage in relieving the soft-tissue injuries of my patients. This is only half true. The name Magic Fingers also comes from my ability to feel and root out the source of the soft-tissue problems, the N-bodies, with my fingers.

I have had my share of unbelievers.

"If I want to get a massage, I'll go to Forty-second Street," said one cynic. "I've never been in a place like this before," a doubting physician stiffly commented. Both changed their minds after they saw and felt the results of my treatments.

I also encounter impatience. People walking into my office for the first time want to get better yesterday. All they know is that it hurts and they simply must walk out being able to do everything they were able to before they experienced the pain.

All the people I work with quickly learn that muscle, tendon, and ligament injuries require more than bed rest or inactivity. To get lasting results from treatment, you have to evaluate the problem, root out the source, understand how to solve it, and take the necessary steps to actively correct it. This can take time.

The focus of this section is on the use of massage to heal problems of soft-tissue injuries.

Every day I average around twenty to thirty vigorous, rehabilitative massages on my patients. Each lasts between thirty and forty-five minutes. It's hard work on my part, and I wouldn't do it if there were an easier, more effective, and less time-consuming way to get people better.

My exposure to tissue-restorative massage as a therapeutic tool began long before I started training in physical therapy. Even in the eighth grade, when I traced the muscles from a kinesiology book, even as I pored over massage books in high school and college, I had a keen interest in the idea of massage as a healing agent. I practiced on friends, athletes, and myself. I later studied with sports trainers from Eastern European countries, who routinely provide their athletes with massage before, during, and after training and competition. Most of all, I have developed my evaluative and treatment techniques through my own experiences as a specialist in manipulation of soft tissue.

However, in order to become a practitioner yourself, you do not need more than a basic knowledge of injuries or of the body in general. What you need is the desire and motivation to learn enough so that eventually you know that by laying your hands on someone you have the potential to help make him or her better.

I have always recommended that the entire family learn massage and regularly work on each other. The more you and others close to you can learn about massage as therapy, the healthier and happier your bodies will be. And as an added benefit, your practice of massage will generally increase the social interactions between family members and friends as well.

If left alone, injuries to the muscles and other soft tissues eventually heal themselves to a degree. However, without massage, or a sensible exercise program, the soft tissue does not return to normal as quickly or as completely. Massage is very easy to learn, and as you will see, improvement is rapid and often dramatic.

In addition to affecting soft tissue, massage also affects the systems of the body, specifically the nervous, circulatory, muscular, and lymphatic systems, and the skin.

Effect on the Nervous System

Massage, when applied properly, uses a smooth, steady, and rhythmical pressure on the body. The effect is a strong hypnotic, relaxing feeling that is not unlike rubbing a baby's back to help him or her to sleep or petting a dog to keep it calm.

When you injure a part of your body, your first inclination is to rub it to soothe the pain. The cause of the injury is irrelevant. You could stub your toe, burn yourself on a hot pot, or bump your knee while getting out of the car. The body's initial reaction to massage is to become calmed down and to experience a reduction of pain. When the nervous system is soothed, the muscle will begin to ease its spasms to a degree. However, in order to break through the tightness, the work must be more vigorous than a calming rub.

Effect on the Circulatory System

During the inflammatory process, blood circulation is increased to bring chemicals to the injured area. This helps to stop bleeding in the area and prevents infection. At the injured site, the cell structure is changed so that fluid normally inside the cell flows out of it into the soft tissue. The excessive swelling causes increased pressure on the nerve endings. The nervous system then directs the injured muscle to tighten in order to limit movement and prevent further injury. The initial inflammation stops when the body realizes that the injury is not a threat, and the goal of the massage becomes a concentrated effort to increase blood circulation to the injured area. More blood going to the injury means more swelling, more nutrients and oxygen, and a removal of waste products from the area.

To give you an idea of why circulation is so important, let's mentally draw a picture of what goes on inside an injured area of tissue. A spasmed muscle can be thought of as a tight fist that is clenched so hard that only limited blood flow can occur. If the tightness of this "fist" is reduced by a calming massage and the muscle begins to relax, it may "open" enough to allow more blood to reach the area. The fist can be encouraged to open more by using greater pressure with the massage. When the fist as tightened muscle finally relaxes, this results in a total improved local metabolism in the muscle.

What's the reason for this? It's because more blood gets to the injury, hence there is more oxygen and lots of healthy nutrients. It sometimes takes weeks of regular massage to get results, but by starting early, the healing process begins sooner, and each session will bring you that much closer to health.

There is a contradiction of sorts here. If all this inflammation, bleeding, swelling, and accumulation of waste products is bad, why do we encourage massage and active movements that are themselves inflammatory? The answer is that sometimes controlled, low-level irritations are necessary as constant reminders to the body to try actively to heal itself. Thus the best way to get rid of soft-tissue injuries is to maintain constant awareness of healing within the body by keeping the "channels" open.

Effect on Lymphatic System

Massage also stimulates the flow of lymph, the clear liquid that helps remove waste products from the body. The flow of lymph and the performance of the muscle depend on each other to function. Therefore, massage becomes very important in encouraging the flow of lymph to areas where pain, illness, or paralysis have stifled the ability of these "cleansers" to remove the waste.

Massage also helps in the case of overactivity. When we overexert ourselves, whether it be a week of "pounding the pavement" with sales calls or a week of advanced aerobics classes, waste products are formed faster than they can be removed. Even in the most favorable of situations, the muscles cannot eliminate the wastes quickly enough on their own. Massage is vital in stimulating the circulatory system to spread lymph fluid efficiently and quickly in order to get rid of the "debris" and restore muscle health.

Effect on the Muscle System

Restorative massage works directly on muscles by stimulating inactive muscles and compensating in part for inactivity due to illness or injury. Deep, continuous massage also relieves muscle tension. A person who counts on Mother Nature for healing will usually return to a certain level, but the N-bodies and waste products will remain rooted in the tissue. Unless they are worked on aggressively through massage, the muscles' aging process begins earlier than it should and the muscles become less reactive.

You can locate problems in a person by feeling the muscles with the tips of your fingers. You can evaluate for muscle tightness by pushing down gently on the affected area and comparing it with the opposite, uninjured side to see if it depresses as deeply. The muscles that cannot be pushed in as far may be tighter.

Effect on the Skin

Skin lives and breathes just like any other tissue of the body. When common functions such as sweating, breathing, and the ability to sense are disturbed by illness, injury, or inactivity, they can be restored by massage.

When Not to Massage

I am extremely progressive in my approach toward massage. Unlike other soft-tissue specialists, I believe in beginning the process immediately. Whenever possible, normally begin massage very shortly after a sprain, strain, or tear.

There are certain conditions, however, when massage is not recommended for treatment. Cancer is a prime example. Because of the possibility of spreading the malignancy to other parts of the body, massage is not advisable.

Circulatory problems of any kind, whether it be high blood pressure or any history of heart trouble, should not be treated by massage. Other conditions that preclude massage therapy as a treatment are: unhealed bone fractures, advanced osteoporosis (if danger of a bone break exists), muscle or bone disease, any skin infections or diseases, severe diabetes, tubercular joints, unhealed frostbite, or burns.

Giving a Massage

Contrary to popular belief, tissue-restorative massage is not supposed to be comfortable. During the first few treatments, a superficial massage is performed to allow the tissues to get used to the new pressures on them, and the person receiving the treatment gradually learns to adapt to the pressure; soon he or she will no longer tighten up during massage.

A deep massage can hurt. Bodies can feel bruised and sensitive the next day or even two to three days after a massage due to minor inflammation of the massaged area. Eventually the tissue adapts, and the bruising stops.

After a few sensitive weeks, I can work more thoroughly on the people I treat. The muscle spasms and tightness begin to disappear, and I taper the frequency of the treatments. The bottom line is that the person feels better and is able to resume a more normal life-style.

I do not stop there. I am never satisfied with having people improve merely to their preinjury level. I want them to be better than they were before.

There are hundreds of massage books on the market today that discuss as many ways to massage. Some offer you techniques with unpronounceable names. Some are too basic, others are too profound, while still others border on erotica. If anything, most massage books manage to confuse beginners, leaving them more intimidated than interested by the procedure. When it comes down to basics, massage *is* basic. There are only three kinds of strokes that you need to know in order to give a strong and healthy rehabilitative massage.

The three strokes are *effleurage*, *petrissage*, and *cross-friction*. If you can master these strokes, especially the different levels of effleurage and friction, you will be as capable as many specialists. Most important, you will have the know-how to accomplish the task at hand, which is simply to make your patient better. Following are explanations of the different massage strokes.

Effleurage

Effleurage can be divided into three different levels of intensity. When you rub, you follow the vertical lines of most of the body's muscles.

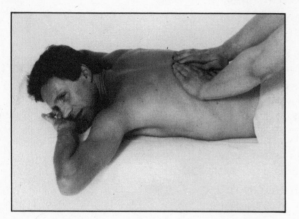

During level 1, use your whole hand, keeping equal pressure on all portions of it. Face your thumbs in the same direction as the rest of your fingers. Push in the same direction that the blood circulates, that is, toward the heart. Keep the strokes slow and continuous, rhythmical, and on the surface only.

For level 2, you put additional pressure on the heels of your hand and you start to press deeper and harder. You advance to level 3 by putting pressure

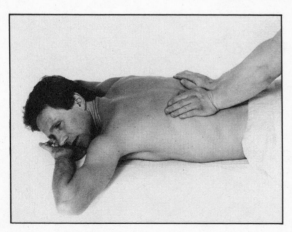

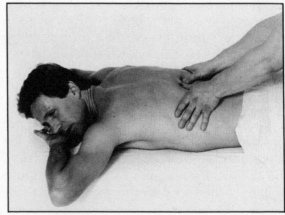

only on the thumbs; this is called *friction*. Here, the
massage penetrates deeper and deeper. The final level, one that your patient may never be ready to handle,
involves what I call "thumb on thumb," where you apply the added pressure of one thumb on top of the other. All the finger positions change during the massage
depending on the depth required and the area to be
treated.

Petrissage

Petrissage involves more of a wringing, grabbing type
of motion. You grab the tissue between the thumb and
fingers and pull it in one direction and then the other.

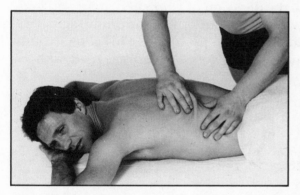 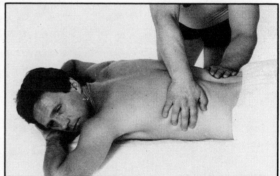

It is similar to kneading bread. I use it more in the stimulating massage, which you will be introduced to later
in this chapter.

Cross-friction

Cross-friction is defined as a deep cross-tissue massage.
When you work on an isolated area, cross-friction is
used at a perpendicular angle to the chain of muscles.

So, if the muscles run up and down, as they do throughout much of the body, friction is used going crosswise. Unlike effleurage, cross-friction does not follow the path of the blood flow. You sometimes push

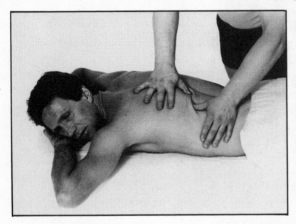 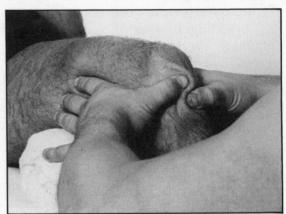

opposite to the direction of your circulatory and muscle systems, pressing hard with your thumb across the muscle and away from the spine. This allows you to smooth out muscle fibers that are clogged with N-bodies.

Massage Equipment

At home, you should set up your working station on top of a desk or a large table. A bed does not provide adequate support, and the floor is too low for the person giving the massage (from now on referred to as the "healer").

Your surface should be arranged so that you can position yourself comfortably with full range of motion. The height of the work station should come to the level of your wrist bones when you are standing with your arms at your sides. If the station is too high or wide, all the pushing power must come from your arms and shoulders. If the station is too low, all pushing will have to come from your back. In both cases, you will get tired a lot more quickly and your massage will be less effective. The proper height of the station allows the healer to work from a balanced stance, using his or her legs, trunk, and arms, rather than just one area.

A six-foot piece of two-inch-thick foam rubber or several pillows or quilt blankets will soften the surface. It is important to have rolled-up towels available for positioning parts of the body in order to relieve pressure.

The temperature of the room must be comfortable, neither too hot nor too cool. Always have sheets or blankets available to drape on the area to keep your subject warm after the massage.

This is important, because during a massage treatment the blood circulation increases in the body. Physical manipulation of the skin causes the skin's pores to open. Upon completion of a massage, the subject's muscles and skin are warmed and if the muscles and skin are not maintained at this temperature for a while, the body will cool off too rapidly. As a result, the therapeutic effects of the treatment will be reduced.

Many different lotions can be used to decrease the friction caused by hand-to-skin contact. Various oils, such as cold-processed peanut oil, mineral oil, or castor oil are good. For people who develop irritation from oil, use hypoallergenic hand cream, and be sure to apply make-up remover or alcohol after the massage. All lotions should be warmed to body temperature before use by rubbing the lotion quickly in your hands, and ideally, the area to be massaged should be shaved for best results.

Now that you have an introductory knowledge of massage equipment and the basic strokes involved, let us evaluate and begin to heal a real subject suffering from a specific soft-tissue injury.

The patient is a young woman named Holly, a physical therapist, who has come to me with a back injury and has been told by two specialists that she has a ruptured disk. She has spent ten weeks in bed to rest the disk on the advice of her doctors. After she became worse instead of better due to inactivity, she came to me in desperation.

As I probe around for the problem with my fingers, I notice several very sensitive areas in her soft tissue, a good distance away from the spine where any problem involving a disk would occur. It is in these tight muscles that she feels spasms so painful that she can barely move. Her problem seems to be caused by poor posture and tension in her body that had finally won out after she awkwardly lifted a heavy patient.

Holly's initial treatments have consisted of restorative massage three times a week. Later, daily exercises are added, which are made increasingly difficult. The massages have also grown more vigorous, though simultaneously less painful for her, since her muscles are now more flexible and in spasm less frequently. Now, two months after her first treatment, Holly is about 85 percent back to normal, the condition her body was in before the injury. In another couple of months, between the massage and the exercise, she will be 110 percent better than she was prior to the trauma. (With disk herniation, it is advisable that patients be monitored closely by their doctors during the course of their therapy.)

Let's take a step-by-step view. I begin by having Holly lie on her stomach across the massage table. She is more comfortable removing all restrictive clothing. She must be draped with towels to keep the rest of the body warm while exposing the area to be treated. You stand behind her on her right (injured) side. You must stand in order to be able to apply the desired pressure.

Begin by working very slowly, using light, rhythmical, somewhat circular strokes with equal pressure from the fingers and palm. (No massage is done totally straight up and down.) Stroke toward the heart in order to encourage blood flow as you continue with your level 1 effleurage. Push harder in your motions going toward the heart than in the ones coming down.

Your hand should begin to conform to the configuration of her body.

Look upon the first minute or two as an introduction to the person you are healing. Your hands will begin to feel the way the person's muscles are shaped and how the patient's back adapts to the first massage strokes. Each of you must get used to the touch, the healer feeling for when the subject's body is relaxed. Stroke up and down along the back, vertical in direction but slightly circular in shape.

Note again that almost all of the muscles in the body run vertically. The major exceptions are the more horizontally-arranged muscles in the stabilizing areas of the body, such as the abdominal area, buttocks, and shoulders.

Continue by gradually increasing the depth of your strokes, advancing to level 2, where you're using the heel of your hand. It's a good idea to draw a mental picture of your hands as though they are actually underneath the skin working the muscle.

Always treat the surrounding areas as well as the injured site. In Holly's case, we massage the right upper leg, buttocks, and lower back, even though her primary injury is in the upper part of her right buttock. The superficial effleurage should relax the uppermost muscles so that the N-bodies can be felt better. Begin to move on to level 3, using three fingers as you move closer and closer to the most sensitive area. Continue to move back and forth from more intense to less intense strokes (from level 2 back to level 1). After a good ten to fifteen minutes of massage, begin using the deep-friction massage, working horizontally to pull the muscles apart and rub out the N-bodies that have formed in the muscle belly.

Do not try to press hard for the first few sessions. Level 3 effleurage, for example, will be too much for many people to tolerate. It takes time for you as the healer to listen and become sensitive to your subject. If you work too hard right away, you can bruise the skin or the muscle tissue. You have to use your discretion here. You must work the body hard to get the desired results, but do not expect to go too deep right away. It may take several treatments.

With Holly, the strokes get deeper and deeper. Yet if I start to feel some resistance, I drop back a level or two. Don't massage at a single intensity, but shift continually up a grade and then down a notch.

Fatigue can be a problem for the healer. To reduce the chances of this happening, you should constantly shift your weight backward and forward on your legs as you massage. You can keep yourself from tiring mentally as well as physically by constantly changing your stroke, along with its level of intensity. Switch every couple of minutes from using your full hand to using the heel, several fingers, or your thumb. Refrain from massaging with your knuckles or your elbows. Both can cause injury if not done correctly.

The beginning healer may physically only be able to massage five to ten minutes the first few sessions, and the subject may be unable to withstand more. After that, with the strokes and levels of intensity interspersed, Holly will get about five minutes each of level 1 and 2 effleurage of the whole back; about fifteen minutes of level 3 effleurage of the lower back and buttocks, her most sensitive areas; maybe two minutes of petrissage for the lower back, for more of a break from routine than anything else; and the remaining time for cross-friction for the lower back. For the final minute or so we return to a more relaxing level 1 effleurage.

While I don't necessarily recommend massage tools, many instruments are available to assist in massage. They are used by soft-tissue manipulators for heavily muscled patients, mostly athletes with a good deal of bulk. They provide rest for a weary thumb.

Although Holly has adjusted to three massages a week, each person will tolerate it differently. Just as it will take you time as the healer to build up from five to ten to twenty and then thirty minutes, it will take your patient time before her muscles or skin can tolerate a deep, restorative massage on a regular basis. Start out twice a week and increase. Eventually, you will be able to do it every day, perhaps alternating days between the normal heavy and vigorous massage, which is necessary to break up the N-bodies, and a light effleurage.

After finishing Holly's treatment, it is best to keep the massaged area warm by wrapping her in a wool or cotton blanket for about thirty minutes. This is to maintain heat from the physical manipulation—you can actually feel the warmth—in the area for an extended period of time.

If the massage has been a vigorous one, Holly may feel somewhat sore. To reduce the inflammation a half hour later, we will apply an ice bag to the area, compressing it with an Ace bandage.

The massage suggestions given here are purely guidelines for technique and positioning. As the healer, you will develop your own methods, and I encourage you to do so. The important part is to start and then continue on a regular basis.

As I mentioned earlier, the best healer is the one who is most sensitive to the needs and feelings of his or her subject. You have to know when to work hard and when to let up. In time, your fingers will become more sensitive to the skin of your subject. You will be able to study the subject's body, aware of where the tight muscles and N-bodies are located. Your fingers will actually be able to "see" for themselves.

To prepare your fingers for working on a subject, you should make them stronger and more sensitive to the touch. You can strengthen your hands and fingers by kneading bread dough, molding clay, using hand grippers, or doing fingertip pushups standing against a wall. Fingers can be made more sensitive by feeling sharp and dull objects of different sizes and textures. Begin touching and feeling square, rectangular, sharp, and dull objects. The idea here is to get your fingers used to feeling. Any sensitivity training you do will make your fingers that much more receptive for healing a patient.

Different Types of Massage

Although the type of massage we have been discussing is primarily for rehabilitation, remember that *restorative massage* is defined as bringing a person back to his or her normal state and does not require that that person have an injury. This could be an active man or woman in training who is more tired after the third consecutive day of intensive exercising than he or she was after the first day. There is no gross physical problem or illness here. Just simple body fatigue.

Instead of working on a localized area, these types of massages are more holistic in that they involve the total body. Soviet therapists, for example, regularly massage their athletes before, during, and after competition—whether the event is weight lifting or swimming. Depending on the desired effect, these treatments are intended either to calm or to stimulate the subject by working primarily on the nervous system.

Slow, rhythmical massage is perfect for someone who has just finished a training session or who has completed a presentation and is too wound up to fall asleep. This soothes and relaxes the body, because blood flow increases to the muscle, so that the nervous system is therefore no longer under as much strain from the muscle tension.

In the case of the athlete training for competition, the massage will bring him back to his original "set point." For example, a runner who put in a ten-mile run on Monday and another on Tuesday is unlikely to be at her same level or set point for training Wednesday unless her fatigued muscles are relaxed and restored by a calming massage. The idea is to soothe the nervous system, as you would by rocking a crying baby. Using the full hand, the strokes are firm but light and always continuous. Ideally, the massage is done in a room with soft lighting and little or no sound.

While this type of massage is usually performed

after an activity, it can also be used to relax a person before he or she competes or gives a speech. Prime examples are a boxer who comes into the ring so keyed up that he forgets his plan of attack, or the public speaker who pales needlessly and wastes nervous energy prior to a presentation. The calming massage relaxes them, preventing them from fizzling out too early. In general, when giving a relaxing massage you're not as concerned about the clinical techniques of the treatment as you are with making the muscles loose, thereby reducing tension.

You can also give a stimulating or "excitatory" massage for those individuals who, instead of becoming hyper before a big job interview or important test, appear listless or distant. This is also the kind of massage that may be given to an athlete who is tired from being overtrained. The stimulating massage involves shorter strokes. The manipulations are short and quick, rather than long and rhythmical. You do some stimulating petrissage rather than low-level effleurage. This massage may last only four to six minutes per body part, rather than the ten to fifteen minutes you do for each body part in the relaxing massage.

The excitatory massage gets the blood pumping into the desired area—whether it be a runner's legs or the neck of someone about to take an exam. Of course, in some cases you don't need a healer; you can give yourself the massage. I did a fifteen-minute stimulating massage on each of my legs before I made my lifetime best lift in the squat exercise.

Massage is a wonderful technique for increasing the health of a local area and for relaxing the body. It relieves pain, decreases certain types of swelling, and helps improve range of motion. Yet, it is only part of the answer. You must spend an even greater period of time exercising to reinforce what the massage has done. While a massage may loosen the area, allow the muscles to contract more efficiently for a longer time without breaking down, or restore them to health, you must keep pushing to raise them to their maximum level of ability and function.

So, all of a sudden, massage takes on a different meaning for us. While you probably once thought of massage as a sensual backrub from a good friend or a loved one, you can see it can be much more. When done properly, massages produce tremendous internal effects that get results.

Over the years, people hearing of my services have said, "Yes, I should get in to see that Marc Chasnov. I don't mind paying for a good massage." My response to these people? If all you want is a nice massage alone, save your money! Getting your body better is a total commitment involving a sensible exercise program *as well as* massage.

Chapter 3
EXERCISE

Exercise and massage share a common purpose—to keep the muscles relaxed, healthy, and ready to perform at all times. However, as discussed before, each part makes up only one-half of your goal: to make the body better. Where massage begins the process of healing, exercise takes it one step further. Massage is the passive treatment, in which the healer manipulates our muscles to root out the waste materials, or N-bodies. Exercise is active treatment, and is crucial not only in getting the body better but in continually improving its performance and condition.

What is exercise? Everyone has his or her own ideas. The captain of the local high school football team may think that exercise is being able to lift three hundred pounds, even if he accomplishes this a single time by muscling the weight up with all his might (and does nothing in the way of a warm-up). Aunt Louise, meanwhile, hits the tennis courts twice a week with her bridge group. Mary, a college coed, jogs two miles every other morning (usually with no more warm-up than a few jumping jacks and leg stretches) and teaches aerobics four times a week. And Harry's idea of exercise is to get up during halftime to stroll over to the fridge for another beer.

Obviously, exercise can be interpreted in many ways! None is necessarily right or wrong. But when you get down to basics and examine a workable definition of exercise, you will learn that there are certain fundamentals that apply to every one of us. The exercises featured in this book are not random movements done a few times each day. Instead, they are a series of organized, natural motions that encourage the muscles to become healthier and stronger, and stay that way.

Exercise is defined as the exertion of muscles to maintain bodily health. It makes no difference if you want to improve your voice quality, eye control, breathing or circulation; all exercises require muscles to use energy in movement. Thus, our first goal in improving any form of exercise is to first develop the muscles.

How Movements Occur

Muscles only move when they are told to move. When the brain talks, the muscles listen. Since the muscles can either contract or relax, the brain must tell them to do so. When muscles are told to contract, they become shorter, and when they relax, they return to their normal position—if they are healthy.

How Muscles Move to Develop Tension

When the brain tells a muscle to contract, oxygen combines with the muscle's "fuel" to cause a muscle to shorten. Thus a muscle contraction is a chemical-mechanical process. The chemicals react with each other and make the deeper, smaller muscle fibers move toward each other. If enough fibers do this, the entire muscle shortens (contracts). When the muscles shorten, tension is produced (as in the bending of an arm or leg). If the tension is strong enough to activate the bones and joints over which these muscles are attached, movement occurs and the bones move closer together. When the muscles relax, tension is reduced and the bones and muscles return to their normal length.

The brain holds many simultaneous conversations with the muscles, telling some to be active and others to be relaxed. This is how all our body movements are created. Our muscles work on the buddy system. If one muscle wants to move, its partner muscles guide and support it to move. If all muscles were to move simultaneously, there would be no control and the movement would be unlimited. By looking at movement from this perspective, it is obvious that the number of possible movements are infinite.

Strength and Work

What makes our muscles work? What gives our muscles the strength to work harder and harder?

First of all, let's define strength and work. Strength is the ability of a muscle to produce tension. When a muscle creates tension and movement occurs, then it is performing work. A muscle may create tension, but does no work if no motion takes place. If the only weight a muscle has to move is the body itself, it can usually accomplish this under normal circumstances. In this case, it is only performing a limited amount of positive work. If additional weight is placed on a part of the body that is moved, then the muscle is performing positive work. Furthermore, the muscle has increased its strength during that brief moment.

Muscles also follow their own rule of supply and demand. If the demand—additional weight or resistance—is greater, the muscle has to supply enough tension (force) to overcome that weight in order to move.

If movements with the extra weight are accomplished regularly and repetitively, the muscle is actively exercising. The muscle adapts to the additional weight by increasing its strength. It is this kind of exercise—a slow build-up of steady, repetitive weight training—that is the foundation of my exercise program.

Exercise does all sorts of good things for the muscles. As the blood flow increases to the deeper layer of the muscle, the temperature of the muscle increases. The warmth makes the muscles function more smoothly and they are therefore more receptive to the signals they receive from the nervous system. Since the muscles require energy to contract, they begin to store up a surplus of chemicals to use for future contractions. The muscle gets stronger and more powerful and moves the bones about a joint as they were created to move. This muscle growth, technically called *hypertrophy*, is a result of an extensive chain of internal events.

History of Massage and Exercise

Massage and exercise are the oldest, most natural forms of treatment used to heal the body. Their use in treating injuries dates back to the priests of ancient China. These priests were among the first people to practice body movement, breathing techniques, and massage in a total, integrated program.

The first organized use of massage and exercise for healing began in ancient Greece during the time of Hippocrates (around 400 BC). In that time, exercise was performed in partially enclosed outdoor areas under the supervision of physical trainers. In addition to exercise, these early Greeks took steam baths, received regular massages, and used swimming pools that had been constructed for physical rehabilitation. Years later, Galen, a Roman physician who was most likely the most prolific writer of medical information of his time, practiced similar techniques in his country. So the idea of using massage and exercise together began centuries ago!

The rapid growth of exercise for health did not really begin until the early nineteenth century. Peter Ling from Sweden, educated in gymnastics and fencing, developed a system that used trainers to provide "activity" programs that consisted of massage and exercise. The exercise program involved "free movement," calisthenic-type exercises that were supervised by trainers. If any resistance (additional weight or pressure) was needed, the trainer provided it manually. These organized massage and exercise sessions developed into what is commonly known as Swedish massage and remedial gymnastics.

Fifty years later, Gustav Zander, another Swedish exercise instructor, invented the first exercise therapy program using machines in conjunction with massage.

The most recent use of active and resistance exercises for healing injuries began in the United States during the early twentieth century. Thomas DeLorme, a physician and weight lifter, introduced his progressive-resistance exercise programs in the 1940s. These programs were used mostly to treat injured servicemen. This was the first documented use in modern times of therapeutic exercises for rehabilitation. Although original and progressive, this program was incomplete in that it did not include massage as one of its basic modalities. This method marked the beginning of the modern era in which the paths of exercise and massage have diverged.

Non-Machine-Oriented Training

It is interesting, and reassuring, to know that for hundreds of years massage and exercise have been used for healing injuries. It has been only in the last twenty to thirty years that this system has been discouraged. As we became a more machine-oriented society, massage and basic forms of exercise were absorbed, lost in the shuffle. Exercise programs nowadays use impersonal computerized machines, excluding hands-on, personalized programs. Massage, which was once considered an integral part of exercise, is now considered a luxury.

The problem with an all-machine approach is that the focus has shifted. Instead of developing better ways of exercising, of using our bodies to strengthen them, we have become obsessed with perfecting the machines.

We prefer running on automatic treadmills and getting a computerized read-out of our heart rate to feeling invigorated from jogging in the woods and enjoying the companionship of a partner. Many seem to prefer high-tech machines to working with a partner in resistance exercises or using basic techniques.

Getting healthier and more fit does not mean having to spend thousands of dollars on clubs and spas where fancy machines, socializing, and looking good are paramount. A better body comes from a very simple commitment to a sensible program of resistance exercises that make you feel good.

There are so many choices of active-resistance training equipment and health clubs. Which are the best—free weights, machines, or combinations of the two? One way to help understand the equipment is to discuss it in relation to the particular area of the body being rehabilitated. For example, let us discuss the differences in the resistance equipment available to strengthen the knee.

The machines use a knee extension device to

strengthen the knee. Most of the major brands (Universal, Nautilus, AMF, Cybex) have these devices. The major differences between the machines themselves are the angles of the seat, adjustments of the seat and foot pieces for individual height differences, and the shape of the cam or pulley on the machine itself. The similarity in function of the machines is that you are locked into position; you do not bear any weight on the body; you are moving only one body part in isolation. Hence, you are using only one muscle group in one plane of motion.

Free weights use the split-squat exercise, which strengthens not only the knee but the hip and ankle as well. It is a multiple-joint, multiple-muscle strengthener. The exercise is done on the ground so that the body is bearing weight. A slight change in the foot position, not possible with machines, will change the orientation and demands of the exercise. Another important fact is that the split squat is a total-body exercise in that it requires balance and support of the upper body while the lower body moves. In point of reference, many other positions in various sports are similar to the split squat. Examples include karate, fencing, wrestling, ice-skating, football, and pitching.

In all fairness, another machine, the leg-press device, is also used to strengthen the hip, knee, and ankle as more of a lower-body unit. But again, the machine does not involve the upright body position or the participation of the upper body.

The split squat is a basic exercise that can be done in the comfort of your own home and is actually better for you than the two other expensive machines. An active-resistance exercise program for strengthening the body should be basic, not extravagant. The goal in using any training equipment, whatever its design, is simple: to strengthen the muscle. Whether your program is focusing on rehabilitation, preventing or correcting injuries, or improving performance, the key elements of your resistance training are the following.

Core Training—Building the Foundation

The core is the centerpiece of the body, responsible for providing support and control for all the other parts. The core includes all the abdominal and back muscles. All functional activities and movements require support from the core. A motion as basic as opening a door requires holding the lower body stationary while the upper body moves to reach forward to twist the doorknob. Developing all parts of the body separately without building the core is like building the framework of a house without a strong foundation.

Harmony—Training the Whole, Not the Part

Some muscles of the body direct motions while others may guide, control, or even oppose them. The body functions best when every part works together as a team. Resistance-exercise training should follow normal movement; that is, all parts should be trained in a coordinated way to affect the whole. For example, the lifting of a grocery bag from a shopping cart to your car is a more complex activity than it would seem at first glance. It requires that the whole body act as a unit to complete the task.

Resistance-exercise training of individual parts is very effective for rehabilitation and sports but should not be considered all there is to training.

Specificity—Simulating the Movement

The activity of transferring the grocery bag from the shopping cart to your car, for example, requires a multitude of movement patterns. You have to bend over, lift the bag from the cart, pivot, squat down or bend over, gently position the bag in the car, and then reverse the entire procedure when you get home.

Training the core and the rest of the body in a harmonious manner will be of great assistance in this activity, but there is nothing like training to simulate the movement as closely as possible. The most appropriate resistance-training exercise to simulate this complex pattern of movements would involve transferring a weighted knapsack from a lower to a higher table, carrying it a certain distance, and reversing the procedure.

The Importance of Correct Technique

Any activity or skill is more effective if it is done right. The exercises have illustrations and photographs accompanying them to encourage correct technique.

Before you plunge into your exercise program, it is a good idea to familiarize yourself with the following definitions:

Muscle strength—the ability of a muscle to develop tension against a maximum resistance one time (1RM).

Muscle power—the rate at which a muscle develops tension.

Muscle endurance—the ability to develop muscle tension for multiple repetitions at a maximum or less-than-maximum level.

Muscle speed—the ability of a muscle to move quickly.

Repetitions—the number of times a movement is performed between intervals.

Sets—the grouping of repetitions separated by a rest interval. For example, one set can consist of six repetitions. You will normally do four to six sets for one exercise.

Guidelines for Beginning Active-Resistance Exercises

You should consider the following points when beginning your program of exercise:

1. Begin with a proper and complete warm-up.

2. Learn the correct techniques of your exercises.

3. Only use resistances when you can still maintain good form. Start off with the lightest possible weight (say one-half pound).

4. Learn proper breathing techniques so that your exercises are more effective.

5. When choosing the order of your exercises, plan on doing the most mentally demanding ones first.

6. Complete each exercise before moving on to the next.

7. Always make sure you allow proper rest time between sets.

8. Be sensible—if your body is fatigued, decrease the quantities for that session.

9. Always include core exercises (those exercises involving abdomen and lower back). This is your key area for all strength building.

10. In any exercise, the last repetition of your last set should be just as dynamic as the first repetition of your first set.

11. Exercise at least three times a week.

12. Never use such heavy weights that the exercise program, which is meant to help you, harms you.

Planning A Resistance Training Program

Every person responds differently to exercise and stress. As a result, a progressive resistance-training program that works for one person's injury may not be effective for another. To accommodate these individual differences, I have used the following training plan as a guideline for healing injuries. This plan has proven successful for me; I know it can work for you.

Follow the guidelines for beginning active-resistance exercises. After familiarizing yourself with the exercises every day for one to two weeks, you will be ready to evaluate yourself to determine your current functional level.

Since the 1940s, the traditional way of testing your immediate strength level was by the one-repetition maximum (1RM) method. The 1RM represented the most weight you could lift using correct technique at your current skill level. Since 1RM requires an all-out effort and could possibly be injurious, a safer variation of the 1RM was devised. For this reason, I use the Relative Repetition Maximum (RRM) method to develop a safer, more controlled training program.

RELATIVE REPETITION MAXIMUM CHART

Repetition Maximum	Percentage of Maximum
1RM	100 (of weight you can handle)
2RM	90
3RM	85
4–6RM	80
7–10RM	70

For example, if you could lift seven to ten repetitions using seventy pounds, this would represent 70 percent of your absolute maximum, which would in this case be one hundred pounds. Instead of lifting one hundred pounds, you would only have to lift seventy pounds seven to ten times. Indeed this represents a safer way to develop your resistance-training program. After establishing your RRM, work within this more controlled situation for two to three weeks to allow your body time to adapt to the new demands placed upon it. After appropriate warm-up, perform 3-5 sets at your RRM per exercise.

In designing your resistance-training program you should first determine your goals. Are you training to return to your activities of daily living or do you want to participate in less demanding sports than before? Do you want to participate in your original sport playing pain-free? Or do you want to prevent future muscle/tendon injuries and improve performance? Whatever level you desire to achieve, you can do so if you follow the Progressive Resistance Exercise Recovery (PRER) chart.

Progressive Resistance Exercise Recovery Chart

Phase	Number of Repetitions	Percentage of Maximum
3	1	100
	2–3	90–99
	4–6	80–89
2	7–10	70–79
	11–15	60–69
1	16–20	50–59
	21–30	40–49
	over 30	30–39

The PRER chart is divided into three phases. Each phase represents a specific level of recovery. Allow two to three weeks in each phase before moving on to the next.

Phase 1 focuses on rehabilitation. The higher number of repetitions with lighter weights is designed to help you familiarize yourself with the exercises and develop good form and full movement while slowly rebuilding the injured area.

Phase 2 concentrates on muscle building to prevent injury and to maintain the strength improvement developed in phase 1. Phase 2 requires moderate repetitions using slightly heavier weights in order to increase muscle strengthening and prevent tissue breakdown.

Phase 3 is primarily used for power building and improvement of performance. The higher levels of weight used here place more demands on your body so that you can accommodate yourself more readily to sports. Accomplishing this phase means returning yourself to your highest sporting level. When tested, your formerly injured areas should have 90 percent the strength of the noninjured areas. You can now return to your favorite sport at your level prior to injury. *Do not stop there!* Return to your RRM chart, test for your new RRM, and return to phase 1 and again work up to phase 3 while you are participating in your sport. This will decrease the chances of recurrence of the injury and allow you to use your skills better.*

*L. Matveyev, *Fundamentals of Sports Training* (Moscow: Progress Publishers, 1981) p. 173.

Chapter 4
RESTORATIVE AIDS

Unfortunately, many people wait until the pain from an injury becomes intolerable before they decide to do anything about it. If you're like most, you have probably twisted an ankle while jogging or felt a twinge in your back when lifting and done nothing about it. But even minor injuries require attention. *All* soft-tissue injuries, regardless of how insignificant they may seem, should be treated immediately by following four basic steps. Think of them as RICE:

1. *Rest.* Stop what you are doing so that you don't make the present injury worse; limit the possibility of further injury.

2. *Ice.* Lower the temperature at the injury site as soon as possible. This reduces inflammation and decreases the amount of bleeding from injured blood vessels within the affected area. The more blood and other fluids that collect at the site of the injury, the longer it takes to remove them and allow the area to heal.

3. *Compression.* Wrapping the area with a bandage reduces the fluid buildup and limits the swelling in the surrounding tissues. Do not wrap the area so tightly that you cut off circulation. You must allow some room for swelling.

4. *Elevation.* By raising an injured body part higher than the rest of your body, fluids will drain away from the area toward the heart, assisted by the force of gravity.

Swelling begins within seconds of the injury,

so don't waste time. Begin the RICE treatment immediately.

Fire and Ice

There has always been a good deal of confusion over
whether an injury should be treated with heat or cold.
Consider the dilemma of the professional athlete. For
many years, baseball pitchers wrapped their arms in
hot towels or applied hot-water bottles after a game
believing this would prevent sore arms. So, many aching arms later, professional trainers and pitching
coaches got wiser. Pitchers today place their arms in ice
after they are finished pitching for the day. This has
become a postgame ritual for pitchers and many other
athletes who use one body part intensively during
training or competition.

Why ice over heat? It makes sense to initially
treat an injury with ice when you consider that one of
the four symptoms of any inflammation is heat. Additional heat applied to the area will result in increased
blood flow to the injured area. If heat is one of the
symptoms of inflammation, then more heat only increases the pain and swelling. In effect, you're putting
heat on heat. As a result, you are further inflaming the
area and making it worse.

This is difficult for many people to understand,
because by applying a hot-water bag or a heating pad
to an injury or by taking a very hot shower, the pain
seems to disappear from the sprained or spasmed area.
You begin to feel better, and the heat is definitely more
comfortable.

In reality, the heat is only working as a temporary "sedative" on the injury. Relief is brief, lasting
only during the time the heat is being applied and for a
short time afterward. Soon enough, however, this
sedative wears off and the pain returns full force, of-
tentimes worse than before.

Exercise and Inflammation

When you think about it, all exercise is inflammatory to the body. By exerting your muscles, you increase blood circulation, create heat, and cause minor trauma. The more vigorous the exercise, the greater the inflammation. In order to achieve a positive training effect, you need to stimulate the muscles by putting stress on them. Since your body is already inflamed from exercise, the heat from a hot-water bottle, a warm shower, or a Jacuzzi simply intensifies the situation and slows the recovery process.

On the other hand, ice cools the area. Just as a refrigerator slows down the spoilage process, ice applied to the body reduces inflammation. It decreases the swelling and stimulates the blood circulation. By doing this, it also reduces the heat in the area and the accompanying pain.

Personally, I have found that the benefits of ice cannot be praised enough. In college, I jammed my knee a day or two before the National Collegiate Athletic Association (NCAA) Olympic Weight Lifting Championships. I could not bend the knee and I was convinced that I would not be able to compete. To treat it, I used ice for thirty minutes on and thirty minutes off the area for as long as I could tolerate it, nearly twenty-four hours. It worked. The swelling went down, the knee unlocked, and I entered the competition with a functional knee joint.

As recommended before, any soft-tissue injury should be treated with ice as soon as possible. There are several ice application techniques, depending on the size of the area to be treated. The ice Popsicle method, otherwise known as ice massage, involves direct contact with the skin. This technique is used for more focused injuries. In this case, a wooden ice cream stick is placed in a paper cup filled with water and frozen. Before use, the paper is removed from the cup and the ice Popsicle is massaged on the injured site.

Extreme caution must be used to prevent frostbite.

Treatment of larger areas involves securing a plastic bag filled with ice to the injury site. Because this technique is static and involves large areas, a thin towel cushion should be used to protect the skin from the ice bag, again to prevent skin injury. A therapeutic ice treatment takes at least ten to twenty minutes. To reduce the chance of frostbite injuries in both techniques, you should have the ice off longer than on. Eventually, as your skin adapts to the temperature change, you will be able to tolerate twenty minutes with ice on and twenty minutes with ice off. Make sure, of course, that the ice is not compressed so tightly that blood circulation to the area is reduced. The injured site has enough trauma without adding the further complication of frostbite.

Although it is not as comfortable as heat, there are athletes who swear by the benefits of ice whirlpools after tough physical workouts. Professional football players have been photographed submerging their bodies in garbage pails filled with ice after practice. Following Soviet sports research, which shows that it takes longer to recover from a workout after a hot shower than a cold one, Russian athletes now finish their training by standing under a chilly spray.

If world-class athletes benefit from the use of ice after workouts, it seems logical that an average person with an injury can be treated the same way. Coaches from the Scandinavian countries take this frigid philosophy one step further. They have their athletes jump into cold streams or snow after training.

I am not suggesting that you dive into a tub full of ice after a tough workout or to relieve the pain of a muscle strain. The difference in temperatures between your body and the ice would probably be too much of a shock. Yet, you can definitely reap long-term benefits by taking a cool shower after your activity, finishing off with a slightly colder rinse. This is a bearable way of rewarding your body after a good exercise session.

Everything you do should be done gradually. This pertains to exercise and massage as well as to restorative aids such as ice and heat. We may look longingly at what people from other cultures do to soothe their bodies, whether it be sitting in hot Turkish baths or jumping into cold streams, and we try to adapt this for our own use. What we forget is that the people who practice these extreme restorative methods have been exposed to them since they were small children. Their bodies adapted to these treatments by the time they were adults. However, when some brave (and foolhardy) souls decide to spend thirty minutes in a 104-degree sauna the first time out or jump into an icy pool of water without building up gradual tolerance for cold water, they may be jeopardizing their health.

When to Use Heat

I do not recommend using heat on a recent injury for at least ninety-six hours, mainly because the inflammation is too acute. If there is throbbing pain, use ice. In fact, whenever you are in doubt, use ice.

It is only later that heat can have a positive, relaxing, therapeutic effect on an injured area. When used at the proper stage, heat will increase blood flow and bring oxygen and nutrients to the area. The water in a warm whirlpool, for example, makes it easier for you to move your body, and the dry heat from a steam bath or sauna will have a soothing effect. In using any form of heat, just be sure that the temperature of the heat (wet or dry) is not too much warmer than your body's internal temperature. Stay away from extremely hot temperatures (anything more than 102 degrees Fahrenheit). Temperatures above this will only worsen the inflammation when applied.

A prime example of this occurs in health clubs all over the country, as people flock to the saunas after exercise. This situation can actually be hazardous to your health. Your body is already well heated from a workout, and as a result your normal body temperature is already increased. By putting yourself into an extreme-heat environment, you intensify the imbalance in your internal temperature. When your body is above 98.6 degrees for any length of time, it becomes more inflamed and you cheat yourself out of a short recovery period.

A perfect example of the dangers of extremes in body temperatures is the marathoner. Some of these runners' temperatures rise to 106 degrees when they are suffering from heat exhaustion, or they can drop to 88 degrees as their systems shut off like a series of switches and can no longer produce any heat. These kinds of situations can be life-threatening.

I'm not saying that saunas should be put on the "must avoid" list. As pointed out before, a sauna provides certain benefits. But, as with all heat, the sauna must be used properly and at the right time. There are a few simple rules to consider:

1. Always cool down after your workout before you enter the sauna. A good way to do this is to take a cool shower.

2. Stay in the sauna for no more than two to three minutes before going back to the shower. Too much sauna time, like too much time under the sun, may result in heat exhaustion. This will only increase your recovery time.

As a rule, heat should never be applied until at least nine to twelve hours after vigorous activity. Only then can it have a truly positive effect on the injured muscle by encouraging blood flow to the area. By the same token, heat should not be used *before* exercising. If applied prior to exercise, the chance of injury may be increased because the body is cooling down as the demand is on the muscles to warm up. A short massage and warm-up exercise will prepare you better than externally applied heat.

Neutral Warmth

I remind my patients to cover their injured areas with a wool scarf or sweater after a massage or exercise (or sometimes even during a workout). Neutral warmth, as it is called, will prevent muscle spasm by using the body's own heat to keep the area warm. Neutral warmth will make you sweat, stimulate blood circulation, and keep the body relaxed. Your body temperature remains at 98.6 degrees or slightly higher, but on the surface it will be warmer.

Topical Heating Agents

Topical agents can be applied to an area in the form of creams and gels to generate warmth. Although I favor neutral warmth for its deeper and more natural effect, most topical agents are harmless and will provide temporary relief for soreness. These products stimulate the nerves to produce antihistamine reactions and are skin irritants, but rarely get deeper than skin level. These skin creams may temporarily relieve your pain, but cannot be considered a satisfactory long-term treatment. Use caution when applying creams and gels *before* activity, since they have a numbing effect that can mask further damage.

Active Rest

The general consensus among health experts these days is that rest is the best answer for injuries and health problems. If you have a cold, go to bed. If you have a serious illness, go to bed. If you have an injury, rest it. The answer is stay still and don't do anything.

Yet, there are many health practitioners, of whom I am one, who believe that an active approach to restoring health is the best path to follow. This philosophy, known as *kinotherapy*,* was originally introduced at the classic European health spas. Treatments at the spas included water treatments in their naturally heated springs, massages, and saunas, along with supervised exercise programs.

This active approach to recuperation in the United States began during World War I, when injured servicemen were kept as active as possible during their rehabilitation. Experience over centuries has shown that the low-level inflammation (fever) of activity, not rest, is important for helping the body heal faster.

When people come to me with an injury, I do not treat them as so-and-so with the injured foot or the aching back. I do not even view them as injured, but instead as individuals who cannot do what they did before their injury. I encourage these people to continue to move as normally as possible; in other words, to take an active rest.

Even if people have a severe back injury, I provide them with exercises they can do in bed, in water, or while sitting in a chair. After all, this loss of health must be considered temporary. People must always be positive and know that eventually they will move, sit, and walk again and that they must prepare for it as soon as possible.

I treat the noninjured areas as well as the injured parts. The injury is healed when the previously injured and noninjured parts work together as one, not simply when the pain is gone.

The same techniques should be used for noninjured and high-level athletes as well. In these cases, active rest allows their muscles to stay healthy, to recover

*T.D. Bompa, *Theory and Methodology of Training* (Iowa: Kendall Hunt Publishing Co., 1983), pp. 91-92.

from strenuous workouts or competition fast, and to give their bodies a total approach to healing.

Sleep and Quiet

The only inactivity I believe in for treating an injury is sleep. First, since it is important to get more than your normal share of sleep when you are suffering from a fever, the same applies when you have an injury. Sleep allows your body to relax. When your body is calm, all your systems can take time out to mobilize their resources to fight inflammation. This is when much of your healing will occur.

Likewise, you should try to limit stress as much as possible during your injury. This is the approach taken by most famous health spas around the world. Their "leave your stresses behind" environment helps speed up the healing process. Unfortunately, since many of us cannot afford a week to bask in luxury, do the best you can by relaxing at home as much as possible. A pleasant atmosphere, a few plants, sharing some laughs with friends in a positive setting—these are the kinds of relaxing things that will help you get better.

Hydrotherapy

Hydrotherapy refers to any exercise performed in water, whether it be the ocean, a lake, or your neighborhood swimming pool. A heated swimming pool is more appropriate for exercising.

The properties of water permit you to be relatively stronger in water than on dry land. In the water, you feel lighter, and there is less pressure on your joints. As a result, you can move more easily and with less pain.

The same exercises discussed for healing the various body parts can be done in water. Resistance can be increased by attaching a plastic paddle to your hands or by using flotation devices or balls.

Water exercises are also for those peole who are afraid of reinjuring themselves. In the water, they can move slowly with less resistance while they build up confidence.

While ice, heat, creams, neutral warmth, exercise, and sleep and quiet provide some sort of effective relief for our aches and pains, these are also ways of reducing your chances of injury in the first place. You should remember that the restorative aids in this chapter are not just "medicine" for when you hurt yourself—they should be used regularly, along with your exercise and massage program, in maintaining good health.

The Chasnov Method at Work

Chapter 5
HEALING

THE SAYING HAS BEEN PASSED DOWN from generation to generation: If you have your health, you have everything. We have all heard this at one time or another, yet we usually take our health for granted —until we suddenly face a situation in which it is jeopardized.

Over the ages, human beings have devoted a good deal of time to finding more efficient ways of making our bodies healthier. Witnessing great developments in the medical field, we have grown to have higher expectations of our health professionals. If we realize that, several years ago, a person completely paralyzed from the waist down faced lifetime confinement to a wheelchair, whereas today a chosen few can walk with the help of computerized electrodes, we say, "If such huge advancements are taking place, there's got to be a better way to get my _____ [you fill in the blank] better."

It's unfortunate that progress in treating soft-tissue injuries has actually been slowed by the advent of ultramodern exercise equipment and fancy therapeutic machines. These have contributed to the reduction of one-on-one personal interaction, so that it is rare today for people to be able to get a hands-on evaluation or to explain their physical problems in detail to a specialist who listens and offers insights about treatment. All too often, high-tech and fast-paced developments have obscured the basics.

I am reminded of a situation that happened

while I was an intern in the physical therapy department of a hospital. I had just completed my first full-tissue restorative massage on a person suffering from a low back injury. Following treatment, the person got up from the table and commented on how good he felt. I was feeling very good about myself for having made that person feel considerably better. A short time later, however, my supervisor, who had observed me, pulled me aside and said, "If everyone in this department spent as much time on patients as you just did, we would never meet our quotas. In this hospital, eight minutes is the maximum for a massage."

My bubble was popped. Here I thought I had done something well and I was being scolded for it! This incident, although disheartening at first, soon became inspirational as I learned that my way was right. Even though massage and exercise weren't used at the hospital, I knew that these two treatments would become the foundation of my healing philosophy.

Thus, the Chasnov Method of restorative massage and exercise came to fruition. First I evaluate, using my hands to determine the degree of the injury. If I find that first- and second-degree tears or strains of soft tissue are evident, they are treatable by my methods. First-degree tears have less than a 10 percent tear in the soft tissue, whereas second-degree tears involve up to 50 percent soft-tissue tearing. Third-degree tears require immediate surgery, but postoperatively require the same therapy as first- and second-degree tears. Once we know that the depth of the injury falls within the boundaries of my treatment, we begin treatment immediately.

How do you use this guide?
To help you identify your problem, all major joints and their immediate surrounding tissue are divided in this chapter into four zones (or circles) with nondefined boundaries. First, you need to determine in which zone of the part (for example, circle 4, or the back part, of the knee) you have pain. Probe with your

fingers to find the N-bodies. Once you locate the problem area—and once you know there is not any fracture of the bone or more serious internal pathology from X ray results—begin your massage and exercise treatment as indicated.

Start with a self-massage or, better yet, have someone else do it for you. Use the guidelines in this chapter until you feel comfortable and confident enough to develop your own massage and exercise program. In order for these massages and exercises to work, you must put them into practice regularly. Remember, you have the power to heal!

At the same time that you have localized and begun massage treatment on one or more of the designated zones, you should begin the specific exercises. There are five levels of difficulty. Gravity-assisted level 1 exercises work with the force of gravity to assist movement. The body is positioned so that the weight of the body part itself moves in the direction that gravity naturally pulls it. To assist in these kinds of exercises, a powder board or support from a partner can be used to guide and control motion. The partner can also help the body part back to its starting position.

In level 2 the body is positioned so that the weight of the body part and the force of gravity have a minimal effect. The only resistance in these exercises is the weight of the body part itself as it is dragged along a supporting surface. The resistance on the drag force to motion (friction) can be reduced by applying "friction reducers," such as talcum powder, on top of the surface. This level is referred to as gravity-neutral.

Level 3 exercises involve using the weight of the body part itself for resistance. Your body is positioned so that the movement of the area you are moving opposes gravity. This is the gravity-resistance level.

As we move into level 4 exercises, we progress toward increasing the weight and resistance of the exercises in the previous level.

Level 5 exercises treat the injured area as a "normal" connecting link of the body. These exercises involve movement that is more demanding than any day-to-day activity and resistances greater than in all other levels.

In levels 1, 2, and 3 and some of level 4, in order to focus on certain body parts, you will need to position your body in one of eight major positions: backlying (on back), prone-lying (on stomach), sidelying (on side), sitting (on a chair), longsitting (legs out straight), kneeling on all fours, half kneeling (upright on knees), and standing.

General Rules for Healing

1. Start Smart

Always start gradually when beginning your program. If you are exercising to get better, you may want to do less repetitions and partial motions of the exercises if the first ones are too difficult, painful, or easily fatigue you. You must be able to complete the full motion of each exercise before you move onto the next level. You should always concentrate on doing the exercises correctly and with control.

2. Treat the Injured Area

To make it easier to focus on healing, I have divided this chapter into "minichapters" by body part. This will make it easier for you to turn to the section that concerns you. As mentioned earlier, each part is divided into four areas, or circles, to help you pinpoint the area of your pain. Even though pain in one area may be "referred" to another area, you will find that you will be able to associate an injury with a specific area and reduce the discomfort and pain in your body without necessarily knowing the exact nature of the injury. The injuries common to each zone are enumerated along with suggested massage techniques and an exercise program for treating the injury.

3. Use Resistance to Strengthen the Injury

In using resistance training for healing an injury, you should begin at your level of ability. For example, if you are at level 3 or below, your main concern is doing your exercises at this level slowly and carefully, concentrating on good technique and higher repetitions to build muscle endurance. You should achieve pain-free full range of motion in level 2 or level 3 before you begin to add resistance at all.

For rehabilitation purposes, if you have more than one injury, you should concentrate on only one or two specific body parts at a time, therefore keeping the actual number of exercises to a minimum. Always work on strengthening the injured area first. After that, you can proceed to exercising the muscles immediately around it in order to support the vulnerable area.

As soon as you can perform a complete range of motion against gravity without pain, you need to find your own repetition maximum (see page 76). Once the strength in the injured area is equal to approximately 90 percent of the uninjured side, you can advance to the next level.

Throughout the entire rehabilitation period, you should be massaging the area regularly and following the information in the restorative section to help you recover for the following day's exercises.

4. Work the Entire Body

It is also important to remember that your whole body is "equal to the sum of its parts." In other words, even though you may have an injury, it is crucial that you view it as one temporarily "bad part" in your body. Too often when we get injured, we tend to isolate the affected area from any activity. Many of us stop exercising altogether.

It is very important to recognize that the exercises in this chapter are designed to make you *use* your injured area (even if only in a limited capacity) and strengthen the areas around it. By doing this, you give support to the muscles surrounding your injury, thus allowing it to heal better and faster.

For example, say your right elbow is injured. You would concentrate on exercising the upper back, neck, and shoulder areas (the supporting areas of the elbow) on both sides, while doing your regular exercises for the elbow itself. Remember, the whole purpose of your program is to take an *active* part in getting yourself back to health!

The early-level exercises in each minichapter are intended to work an injured zone, while the higher-level exercises strengthen all the other zones surrounding the injury. Most important, this is a self-paced program. There is no time limit, and you can build at your own speed. For example, your first massages may last no more than five to ten minutes, three to five days a week. It takes time for you, as either a "patient" or a soft-tissue healer, to get to the point where you are able to give or receive thirty minutes of vigorous massage.

So now that the rules are set and the guidelines laid out, where do you start? In the exercise section, many active people will be able to begin right away with level 3. Older and more disabled individuals might have to begin with levels 1 or 2. If this is too much, you can start by working out in a pool (see "Hydrotherapy," page 87).

Also included in each minichapter are case histories of people I have treated. The examples show how improper evaluation, diagnosis, and treatment can prolong pain and loss of function from an injury. Take particular notice that many injuries are soft-tissue injuries that respond to the Chasnov Method.

The Neck

The neck is one of our most vulnerable joints. After all, it connects the head to the rest of the body! When you compare it to the two stable, fixed body parts it holds together (the head and the chest), the neck is extremely flexible. It is this very freedom that makes the neck so vulnerable to injury.

Picture the neck as a spring between the head and the chest. In the human structure, this spring is arched forward. The slight arch allows any downward

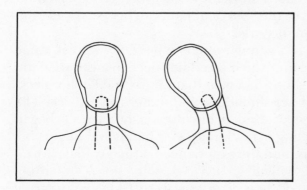 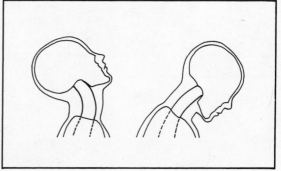

force on the head to be absorbed by the neck without excessively compressing the spring. Without this arch, a blow to the head, for example, would not be cushioned.

Generally speaking, the more mobile a region

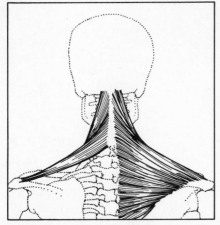

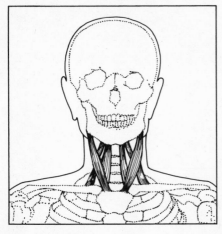

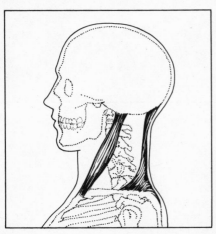

of the body, the greater the amount of muscle and soft-tissue support in that area. In the neck there is a large "support staff" of muscles, tendons, ligaments, and other soft tissue, as well as seven neck bones and the disks between these bones.

The primary shock absorbers are the muscles, tendons, ligaments, and other soft tissue. The secondary shock absorbers are the disks or intervertebral tissue. The last area to absorb shock is the bones themselves. When the body is put under stress, the shock is cushioned in that order. It takes a great deal of force for the body to resort to its third line of defense, the bones (which would result in fracture), so damage to the soft tissue is much more common.

If tests reveal no fracture or ruptured disk you should begin the Chasnov Method immediately.

N-bodies are prevalent in many areas of the neck. They can be loosened manually through massage.

Since so many nerves are situated in the neck area, problems that originate there may actually be felt in other areas—the jaw, up to the head, to the middle back, shoulders, down the arms, and even to the hands. Examples of this source of pain can be seen by the following case histories:

Jody, a young woman in her late twenties, came to see me after she injured her neck in a car accident. Originally Jody had pain that was focused in her neck, the top of her shoulders, and in her upper back. The original pain subsided, but after six months she began to lose feeling in her hands. Her hands and fingers became weak, and she experienced difficulty in performing simple activities, such as opening doors and lifting her child. Jody was diagnosed as suffering from carpal tunnel syndrome, a disease process specific to the wrist and hand.

By the time she came to me, she was scheduled for surgery on both wrists. During the evaluation, I saw that she did not have the standard muscle weakness and loss of feeling in her hands and fingers characteristic of carpal tunnel. However, as I felt her neck and upper back on both sides, I found a large buildup of N-bodies that were possibly compressing her nerves. I immediately gave her a program of massage and exercise. Eight to twelve weeks later she was pain-free and fully functioning—without surgery.

John, an active man in his mid-thirties, is a literary agent who spends ten to twelve hours each day hunched over manuscripts. As a result of the demands of his job and his generally poor posture, John's shoulders were rounded, the area around his cervical spine arched and his head thrust too far forward. The pressure on his neck muscles from the tension had become steadily more painful over the past five years. He saw me after failing to find relief from other health professionals, who told him he had maladies ranging from arthritis to a cervical disk problem to a pinched nerve.

My evaluation revealed N-bodies and tightened, imbalanced muscles in his neck. I told him that we could reduce and possibly eliminate the pain after a program of regular massage and a gradual buildup of exercises within twenty-five sessions. On the day of the twenty-fifth session, John said, "Guess what?" and walked out of my office without any pain.

One of the more shocking evaluations was of Sam, a marathon runner in his late forties, who was experiencing crippling neck pain. After multiple neurological tests, one health professional told him his problem was ALS, or amyotrophic lateral sclerosis, commonly called Lou Gehrig's disease. This fatal neurological disease causes the progressive deterioration of body tissues. The diagnosis understandably scared Sam out of his wits. He consulted another physician who told him that he had severe chronic arthritis. I discovered, however, that Sam simply had extremely tightened muscles and N-bodies in his neck from poor posture that resulted in spasms and compression of the nerves. After thirty sessions, he was running again pain-free.

Tracy came to my office complaining of headaches, dizziness, and pain down the back of her head, neck, and shoulder blades. She was told by her dentist that she had temporal mandibular joint (TMJ) syndrome, a problem resulting from alignment problems where the jawbone meets the skull. She had tried mouthpieces, braces, nerve stimulators, and had even had some of her teeth filed down before she met me. Manual evaluation revealed N-bodies in her jaw and skull area, as well as in between the shoulder blades, in the neck, and on the back skull-bones. Deep massage and exercise relieved the problems she had experienced for three years.

Joan, a woman in her late forties, had contracted polio as a six-year-old. She wears leg braces and walks with crutches and had never exercised her head and neck. She was told she had postpolio pain syndrome, and to relieve the pain she was given heavy medication, acupuncture, and biofeedback. I began working with her, giving her deep-tissue massage and exercises. After forty sessions, she says she hasn't had so little pain in the past seventeen years. While she may never become totally pain-free, her progress has been dramatic.

As different as their situations are, all of the people just mentioned came in for soft-tissue evaluations that revealed N-bodies, weak neck and upper-back muscles, and poor head, neck, and shoulder posture. All too often, people come to me after having been told to rest, take medication, and/or advised that they need surgery. Sometimes they come in wearing immobilizing neck braces. In many cases, there has been little or no improvement with these treatments. Cases once diagnosed as pinched nerves, subluxed vertebrae, and whiplash have responded well to my program of massage and exercise outlined here.

The major goal of this treatment is to reduce the spasm of the soft tissue by massage and exercise, allowing the head and neck to return to normal (or better) alignment and to strengthen the supporting muscles in order to reinforce the alignment.

Massage (Sit with head resting on a pillow on a table.)

1. Spread cream or lotion over the upper back and neck area.

2. Begin massaging with superficial effleurage. Work in a triangle by massaging with both hands in an upward vertical motion from the upper back to the neck, out to the shoulders, and then back down again.

3. Now do a deeper effleurage. Working this same triangular area, use the heels of both hands to go deeper. You can also alternate, using the heels of your hands with the first three fingers of each hand.

4. Start petrissage. Working deeper over this same area, use the thumb and fingers of both hands to grab and pull the tissue.

5. Massage even more deeply, performing friction by using both thumbs to make small circles on either side of the spine, working upward from the upper back to the bony prominence at the back of the head.

6. Using both hands, follow the friction with a deep effleurage to help soothe the tissue.

7. Repeat the petrissage upward over the triangular area, concentrating on both sides of the neck.

8. Do a deep effleurage over the same area.

9. Finish up with a light effleurage, using your whole hand.

Exercises

(Flexion and extension exercises should be performed for problems involving the soft tissue in the front and back of the neck. Lateral and rotational motions should be done for injuries to either side. Before attempting level 4 or 5 of this program, refer back to the guidelines on page 93.)

Neck Flexion

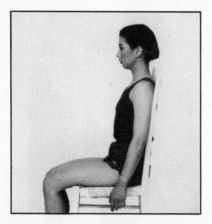
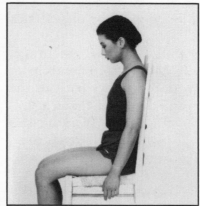

Level 1:
   Sitting or standing, tilt your head and neck down.

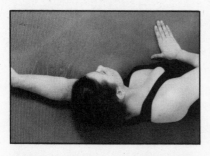
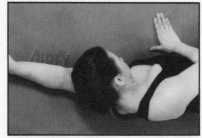

Level 2:
   Lie on your side and bend your chin toward your chest.

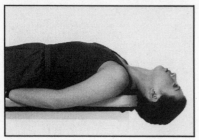
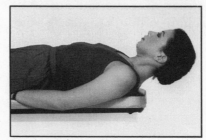

Level 3:
   Lie on your back with your head and chin unsupported over the edge of a bench. Move your chin toward your chest.

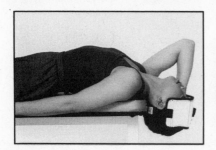
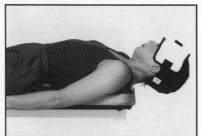

Level 4:
   Same as level 3, adding resistance by strapping a weight around your forehead.

Level 5:

a. Lie on your back with your head unsupported over the edge of a bench and turned toward one shoulder. Lift your head toward the other shoulder. Do the same for the other side.

b. Same as preceding exercise, adding resistance, as in level 4.

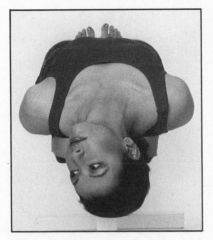
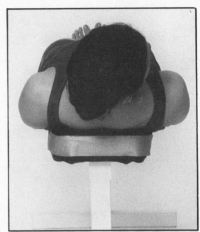

Neck Extension

Level 1:

Lie on a bench on your back with your head suspended over the edge (head may be supported by a partner). Move your head back.

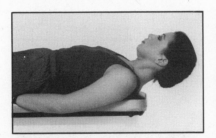
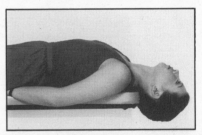

Level 2:

Lie on your side with your head supported by your arm. Move your head back.

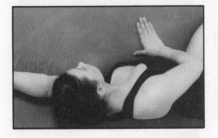
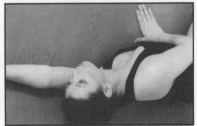

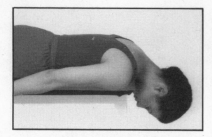
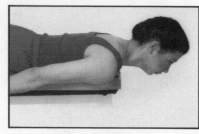

Level 3:
Lie stomach-down on a bench with your head and neck hanging over the edge. Lift your head up.

Level 4:
a. Same as level 3, adding resistance.

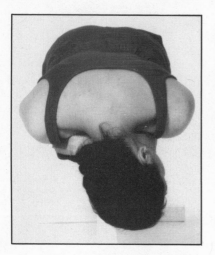
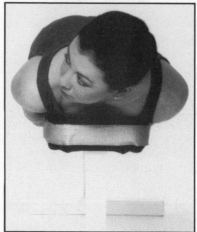

Level 5:
Lie stomach-down on a bench with your head bent downward toward your right shoulder. Lift your chin up over your left shoulder. Do the same in the other direction.

Lateral Neck Flexion

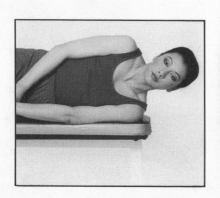
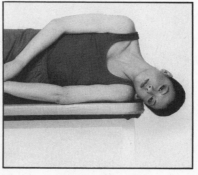

Level 1:
Lie on your side on a bench with your head suspended over the edge and, while supported by a partner, let your head drop toward the floor.

Level 2:
Lie on your back on a bench with your head suspended over the edge and move your head to one side, back to the starting position, and then to the other side.

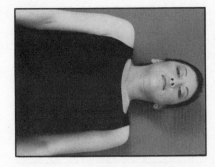
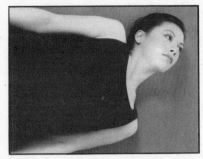

Level 3:
Lie on your side on a bench with your head hanging unsupported over the edge. Lift your head up toward the ceiling.

Level 4:
Same as level 3, adding resistance with a weight or cable.

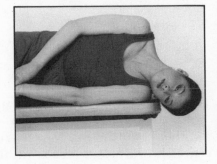
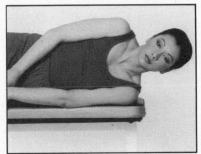

Neck Rotation

Level 1:
Lie on your back and turn your head first to one side and then to the other.

Level 2:
Same as level 1, either sitting or standing.

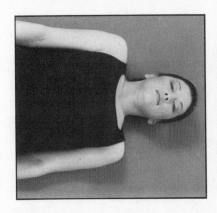
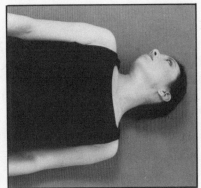

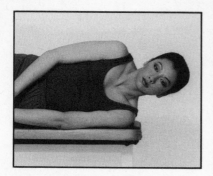
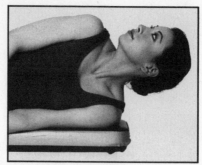

Level 3:
Lie on your side with your head unsupported over the edge of a bench and turn your head upward. Do the same on the other side.
Level 4:
Same as level 3, adding resistance.

The Shoulder

The shoulders are the most mobile joints in the body and the only body part that can rotate 360 degrees (other than the hip joint). With this freedom of motion, however, comes a natural instability. Many shoulder problems are due to irritations of the muscles; the tendons, which connect muscles across the joint to the bone; and the bursas, which lie underneath the tendons and are small, jellylike sacs that prevent the tendon from rubbing against the bone.

Jane came to me with tremendous pain in her right shoulder that she had been told was tendonitis. Rest was recommended. As a result of her pain and the lack of movement from the splinting of the arm joint—Jane couldn't snap her bra strap or lift her arm up without also moving her whole shoulder and forcing her entire body to lean over—I was convinced that what might have begun as a simple tendonitis had turned into adhesive capsulitis (or frozen shoulder).

This injury involves a tightening of the sleeve-like structure that holds the ball and socket of the joint together. This tightness in the area in turn prevents movement. Simply by feeling Jane's shoulder, I noticed that the soft tissue was as hard as a rock on the bad side compared with the soft texture of the muscles and tendons on the good shoulder. Although the joint capsule itself cannot be massaged effectively, there was plenty of N-body formation in the shoulder muscles and tendons. In addition to a deep massage and exercise program, I gave Jane a series of special stretching exercises to gradually restore her shoulder area to full movement.

A frozen shoulder takes longer and is more difficult to treat than a simple tendonitis, in which the person may have pain when moving the shoulder in different positions but still has a full range of motion. This again is best treated by massage and exercise.

Arlene, who came to me with throbbing shoulder pain, had been diagnosed as having a dislocated shoulder. An active woman in her fifties who regularly played tennis, she had to stop playing altogether because of the pain. During the evaluation, I found that the front of the shoulder joint was unstable from a lack of muscle support. Because the areas surrounding her shoulder were not strong enough, extra demands had been placed on the shoulder tendons.

When I mentioned this to Arlene, she wondered out loud if this lack of muscle support could be the result of the modified mastectomy surgery she had undergone years before. The operation had removed muscles in her chest and around her underarm, as well as her breast. The area had since atrophied, placing all the burden of movement in swinging a tennis racquet on her shoulder tendons.

Before we started treatment, we had to be sure that Arlene was out of any danger of a cancer recurrence, as my treatment could be harmful if she were not clean of the cancer. Arlene was referred to me with a medical clearance so I began to massage the inflamed area to get rid of the large N-bodies that had formed there. I also gave her an exercise program to strengthen her shoulder and chest.

Most of the more common shoulder injuries are caused by overusing the muscle/tendon. Baseball pitchers and tennis players (and anyone else who puts a great deal of strain on his or her arms and shoulders) are prone to tendonitis of the bicep, tricep, deltoid, and supraspinatus (the muscle along the top of the shoulder blade) as well as to strains within the rotator-cuff muscles, which are the four muscles and their tendons that hold the ball and socket of the shoulder joint together in the rear of the joint. Tenosynovitis, another shoulder injury, is a localized inflammation of the bicep tendon and its sheath in the front of the shoulder.

A complete or partial shoulder dislocation is also common among active people. (Repeated episodes of shoulder dislocation are not normal, however, and can lead to destruction of the normal bony architecture and soft tissues. An orthopedic evaluation is necessary.) What happens in this case is that the upper arm bone is pulled out of the socket for a brief time, although the muscles in the front of the shoulder may be strong enough to keep the ball from coming out completely. Regardless, the tendons become extremely irritated and need to be made healthy again.

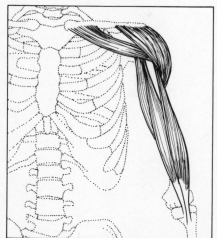

Areas of Common Injury

Circle 1 - (front) Common soft-tissue injuries: bicep tendonitis, bicep tenosynovitis, muscle strain, shoulder separation, shoulder dislocation, referred pain from nerve compression (see neck). Exercise: shoulder flexion

Circle 2 - (side) Common injuries: supraspinatus tendonitis, deltoid muscle strain, shoulder separation, strain in the trapezius muscle. Exercise: shoulder
abduction

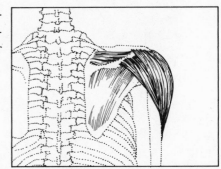

Circle 3 - (back) Common injuries: rotator-cuff
injuries, tricep tendonitis, trapezius muscle strain. Exercises: shoulder extension and outward rotation

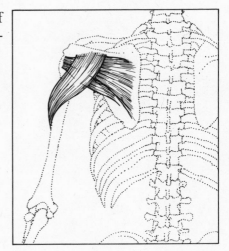

Circle 4 - (underneath) Common injuries: muscle and tendon injuries to the muscles in tricep, lattisi-
mus, and chest-muscle area. Exercises: shoulder
inward rotation, adduction, flexion, extension

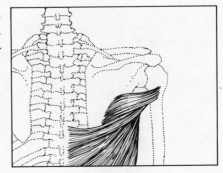

Massage

1. Sit with your shoulder and arm resting on a table.

2. Spread cream on the shoulder and upper arm.

3. Start with superficial effleurage, using both of your hands and massaging from the arm upward to the shoulder.

4. Now do a deeper effleurage. Alternate using the heels of your hands with the first three fingers of both hands, in deep, steady strokes, massaging from the arm upward to the shoulder.

5. Begin petrissage. Use the thumb and fingers of both hands to grab and pull the tissue in a kneading motion, similar to kneading bread, working from the arm up to the shoulder.

6. Now use friction to massage much deeper. Use just your thumbs in crosswise patterns to work at the injury, going as deeply as tolerated.

7. Follow friction with deep effleurage.

8. Now repeat petrissage again.

9. Repeat deep effleurage again.

10. End with superficial effleurage.

Shoulder Flexion

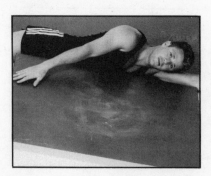 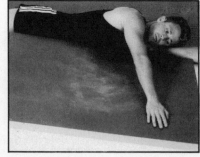

Level 1:
Lie on your side with your arm resting on the peak of a board angled down toward your head. Move your arm along the board until your arm is overhead.
Level 2:
Same as level 1, keeping the board level.

Level 3:
    Sitting or standing, lift the arm up.

Level 4:
    Same as level 3, adding resistance with weights.

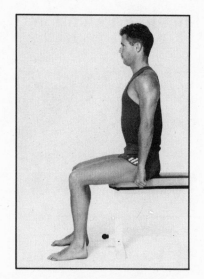
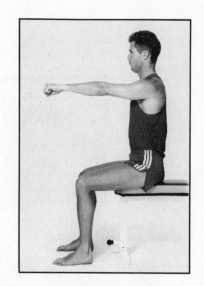

Level 5:
    a. Incline presses— Lie on an incline board, holding a weight, such as a dumbbell, in each hand. Starting with the elbows bent, lift the weights straight up overhead.

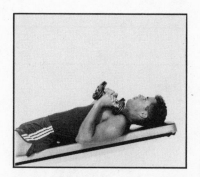
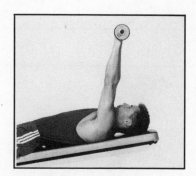

    b. Bench presses— Same as incline presses, lying on a level surface instead of an incline board.

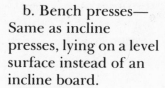
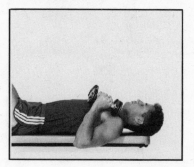
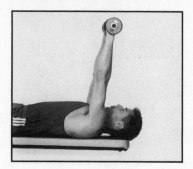

Shoulder Extension

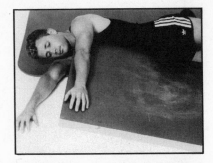
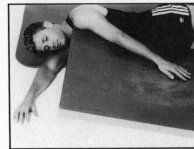

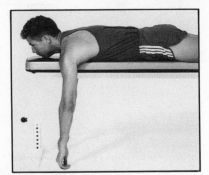
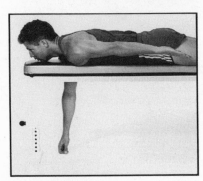

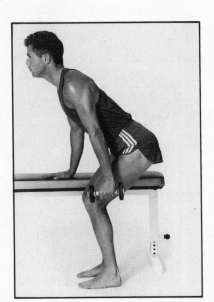
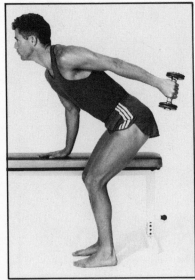

Level 1:
Lie on your side with arm resting on the peak of a board angled away from your head. Move your arm down the board toward your body.

Level 2:
Same as level 1, keeping the board level.

Level 3:
Lie stomach-down on a bench with arms hanging over the edge. Lift each arm backward toward the ceiling.

Level 4:
Same as level 3, adding resistance with a weight or cable.

Level 5:
Bend over a table, supporting yourself with one arm. Move the other arm back, using a weight or cable as resistance.

Horizontal Flexion

Level 1:

Sit with your arm resting on the highest point of a declining board and your elbow bent. Move your arm across your chest in the direction of the decline.

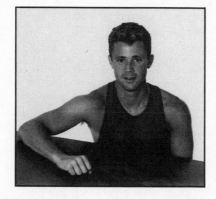
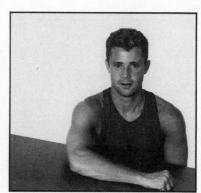

Level 2:

Same as level 1, with arm resting on a level surface.

Level 3:

Lie on your back with your arm out to the side and your elbow bent at 90 degrees. Move your arm across your chest toward the other shoulder.

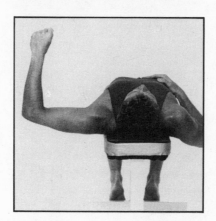
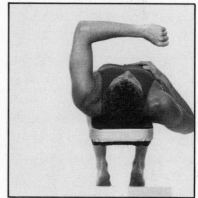

Level 4:

Same as level 3, adding resistance by holding a weight in your hand.

Level 5:

Cable Crossover— Holding either one or two cables (one in each hand), move your arm(s) horizontally across your chest.

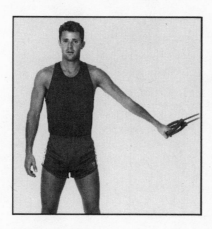
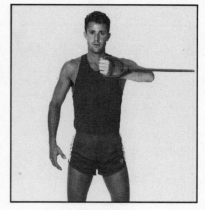

Horizontal Extension

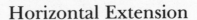

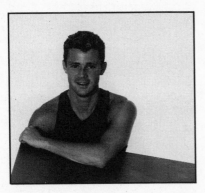 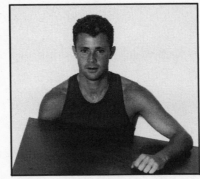

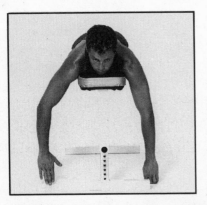 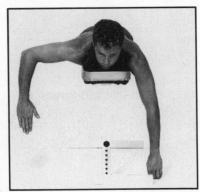

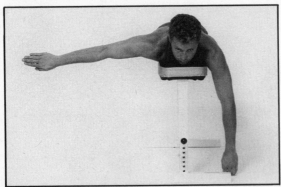

Level 1:
Sit with your arm resting on the peak of a board that declines from the opposite shoulder. With the elbow bent, move the arm down the board.

Level 2:
Same as level 1, with your arm resting on a level surface.

Level 3:
Lie stomach-down on a bench and let your arms hang over the edge. Lift your elbow until the arm forms a 90-degree angle and then straighten the arm out to the side.

Level 4:
Same as level 3, adding resistance with a weight.

Level 5:

Lie stomach-down on a bench and hold a stick with both hands. Draw upward to simulate a rowing motion.

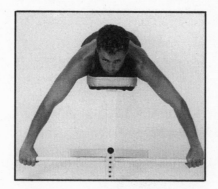
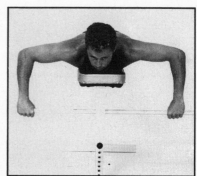

External Rotation

Level 1:

Lie on your back with your arm out to the side and your elbow bent at 90 degrees so that your hand points to the ceiling. Move your hand back to the floor toward your head.

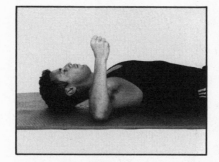
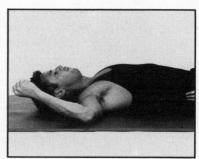

Level 2:

Sit with your arm bent, supported by a bench. Move your forearm back, pivoting on your elbow.

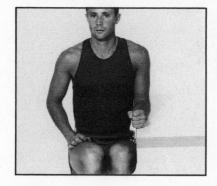
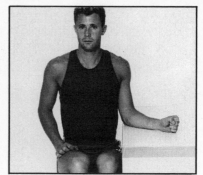

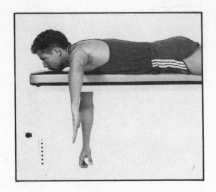

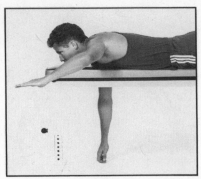

Level 3:
Lie stomach-down on a bench with your arm out to the side and your forearm hanging over the edge. Lift your hand up toward the ceiling.

Level 4:
Same as level 3, adding resistance with weights.

Level 5:
Stand with your arm at your side and your elbow bent at 90 degrees. Supporting your elbow against your side, pull against a resistance, such as a cable, away from your body.

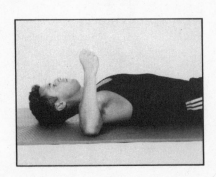

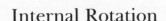

Internal Rotation

Level 1:
Lie on your back you your arm out to the side and your elbow bent at 90 degrees so that your hand points to the ceiling. Move your hand down to the floor toward your feet.

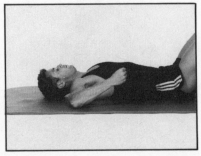

Level 2:

Sit with your arm bent, supported on a bench, and your hand pointing to the side. Move your forearm forward, pivoting on the elbow.

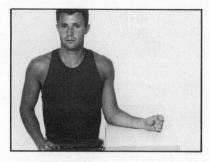 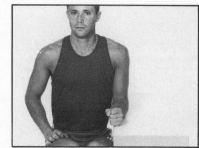

Level 3:

Lie stomach-down on a bench with your arm out to the side and your forearm hanging over the edge. Lift your hand back toward the ceiling.

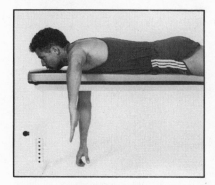 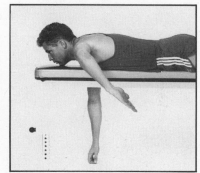

Level 4:

Same as level 3, adding resistance with weights.

Level 5:

Stand with your arm at your side and your elbow bent at 90 degrees. Supporting your elbow against your side, pull against a resistance, such as a cable, toward the center of your body.

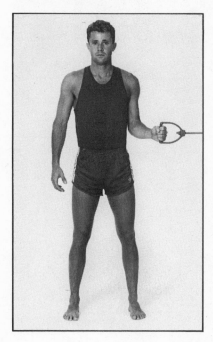 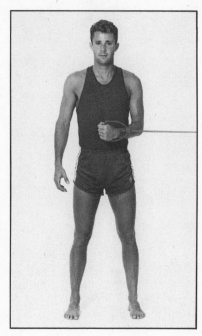

Abduction

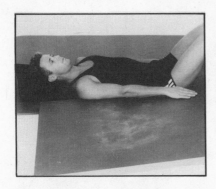 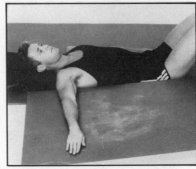

Level 1:
Lie on your back with your hand on the peak of a board declining toward your head. Move your arm down the board.

Level 2:
Same as level 1, with arm on level ground.

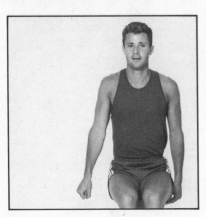 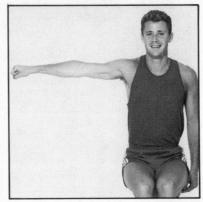

Level 3:
Sitting or standing, raise your arm out to the side to 90 degrees. Do with arm both straight and bent.

Level 4:
Same as level 3, adding resistance against weights.

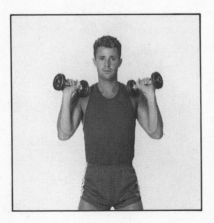 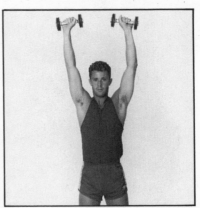

Level 5:
Power Jerks—Holding dumbbells at shoulder level, with knees bent, lift weights straight up overhead in one motion.

Adduction

Level 1:

Lie on your back with your arm out to the side on the peak of a board declining away from your head. Move your arm down the board to the side of your body.

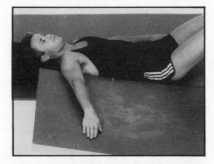 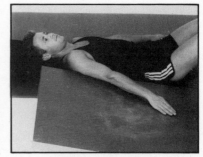

Level 2:

Same as level 1, with arm on level ground.

Level 3:

Standing, hold a cable at a 90-degree angle to your body. Pull the cable down to your side.

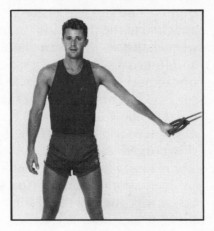 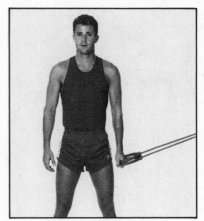

The Back

The Upper and Middle Back

While I don't want to reiterate the basic function of the back, described in "Building the Foundation" (page 16), it is important to take a general view of the back before discussing a healing program.

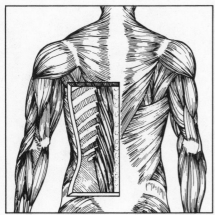

The upper and middle back are both included within the twelve thoracic vertebrae. These vertebrae received their name from the area they support, the thorax. The ribs are located within the thorax and are attached to the thoracic vertebrae. They protect the inner organs, act as external attachments of the muscles, and internally they provide an attachment for the diaphragm, the primary muscle in respiration.

The curve in the thoracic region is arched backward to allow for the extra space occupied by the ribs and internal organs. Of the four curves of the spine, this curved area has the largest number of bones. Therefore, it is a fairly stable area. The majority of problems come from postural habits that, when combined with the increased forward arch in the neck and lower back, cause the backward rounding of the thorax. An overall imbalance results, and the muscles in the rear shoulder-blade area cannot support the weight of the chest. It is as if too much weight were being put on a shelf and the shelf began to tilt and pull out from the wall.

Poor posture is a lifelong erosion process that is primarily caused by poor movement habits and lack of proper exercise during childhood. Once the tendency for poor posture begins, changes occur in the muscles and bones. All muscles are weakened: Some stretch, others shorten, but both become temporarily fixed in the tightened position. The muscle imbalances cause the bones to realign, sometimes pushing them closer together. These structural changes cause pressure on the blood vessels and nerves and the spine itself. Prolonged inflammation will cause N-bodies to develop.

In the area of the middle back, the nerves start in the back but circle around the front to end up in the chest and abdomen. An injury or constant posture strain can cause pain to be referred to those areas.

Debbie, who had pain that traveled into the back of her arms, her neck, down the side of her body, and the front of her chest, was concerned that she might be having a heart attack. Fortunately, tests revealed that her heart was pumping fine. The problem turned out to be some very tight muscles near the spine. After several months of treatment on her middle back, she was feeling no pain.

But the problem can get worse. As the ribs are pulled down, the collarbone and the shoulders "slump" as well. When the shoulders round, the shoulder blades are pulled sideward and up, away from the ribcage. The effect on the soft tissue is that the muscles that hold the shoulder blades together are placed under constant tension. They develop N-bodies and associated muscle spasms that reinforce the problem.

Marie, a runner, came to me complaining of pain that originated between her shoulder blades and would spread into her neck, shoulder, and back of her arm, with a greater problem on one side. She had been told that the problem was a degenerated thoracic disk and that one of her disks was subluxed and out of alignment. She had tried various types of treatment— traction, manipulation, hanging upside down, acupuncture—none of these methods did a thing. Deep massage worked out the N-bodies in the muscles between the shoulder blade and spine. Exercises were performed to improve the posture of the ribcage.

The Lower Back

The lower back is that part of the body that connects the ribcage to the pelvis. The mechanics of this area are very similar to those of the neck. Remember the two fixed objects connected by the spring? In the case of the low back, the upper fixed object is the ribcage and the middle back and the lower fixed point is the pelvis. Again, the spring consists of vertebrae, cartilage, muscles, tendons, and ligaments.

One major difference between the mechanical comparison of the neck and the lower back is that the back has a much greater burden to carry. The lower back has to absorb the extra weight of the head, neck, ribcage, upper and middle back, and all of the internal organs. The muscles of the lower back are much larger and thicker than those in the neck in order to support this extra load. The abdominal muscles may account for up to 40 percent of this support. In the neck, the strength of the muscles in front of the spine provided support.

As with the neck, the large number of nerves traveling from the low back down to the legs may result in pain in the groin, buttocks, hips, back of legs, knees, and down to the shins and feet. The following examples will help explain this:

Bob, a businessman in his early forties, came to me with pain in his lower back that shot down into one leg. The area was numb and weak, and every time he ran or bicycled, he said it felt as if the leg would go out on him. Like most people with chronic pain, he had made the rounds. Treated for two years with rest, medication, traction, manipulation, injections, and acupuncture, Bob's injury was still no better. Upon examination, I found N-bodies from the gluteal fascia, the area above the buttocks, all the way down to the top of the iliotibial band (along the outside of the thigh). It took no more than a dozen sessions of massage and exercise before he was free of all discomfort.

Candice had spent weeks in bed taking anti-inflammatory drugs after the severe pains in her lower back that ran down to her foot. It left her all but incapacitated. A singing instructor and a regular at a local aerobics class, Candice's active life had been greatly changed by an injury whose source she could not even pinpoint (which is often the case with a lower-back injury). Evaluation revealed N-bodies on the crest of her pelvic bone. I started treating her three times a week with deep massage and exercise. Within two months, she was back to normal.

I have had patients who have been told that they have degenerated disks, compressed disks, lumbago, rheumatism, low-back derangement, pinched nerves, sciatica, and arthritis.

There have been instances where the injury was not only to soft tissue but involved the second-degree shock absorbers, the disks. In those cases of true herniation, although the disk cannot always be healed with the Chasnov Method, the soft tissue around it can be treated with massage and exercise to strengthen the area and reduce the pain. Exercise is the most important component, regardless of the disability. Like other parts of the body, all the muscles surrounding the lower back must be strengthened in order to get the support you need.

The goals for treating the lower back are similar to those for the neck. The low-back muscles have to be stretched in order to decrease the forward curve and to line up the ribcage over the pelvis. Once the area is elongated, all of your abdominal and lower-back muscles have to be strengthened to maintain the correct alignment. Due to the increased size of the lower-back muscles, more force is needed to stretch and strengthen these muscles than most specialists realize.

As with any back problem, the more weight carried in the abdomen the greater the pressure on the injured area. It is no mere coincidence that heavy men and women are much more prone to back pain. Therefore, abdominal-strengthening exercises are very important and should be performed hand-in-hand with the exercises for the back once the patient is on his or her way to recovery.

Massage (Lie on stomach with pillow under pelvis.)

1. Spread cream over the entire back.
2. Begin with superficial effleurage, massaging upward from the lower to the upper back. Use both hands in a long, vertical motion.
3. Now do a deep effleurage over this same area using the heels of both hands to massage the tissue more deeply. You can also use the first three fingers of both hands to alternate with the heels of your hands.
4. Now do petrissage, working from the lower back to the upper back.
5. Start friction massage, moving both thumbs in a deep, circular motion up along the back. Do one side of the back, then the other.
6. Continue friction massage using both thumbs in a deep, horizontal sliding motion. Working one side of the back at a time, begin at the low back and slide one thumb away from the spine, and the other thumb in toward the spine. Continue alternating your thumbs as you work your way up the back.
7. Now do a horizontal, deep effleurage across the lower back. Starting on the outer sides of the back, use the heels of both hands to massage in toward the spine.
8. Follow with a three-point upper-back massage to work the trapezius muscle. Massage one side of the upper back at a time. First use the heel of one hand to stroke from the middle of the back up to the neck. Second, use your other hand to stroke from the neck outward to the shoulder. Third, stroke with the heel of your hand from the shoulder back down to the middle of the back.
9. Repeat petrissage, working both sides of the back.

10. Repeat friction, placing one thumb on either side of the spine and making small, deep circles moving from the lower to the upper back.

11. Repeat deep effleurage, now using the heels of both hands.

12. End with a superficial effleurage.

Exercises

<u>*Level 1:*</u>
Sitting, push yourself back into a cushion or ball.

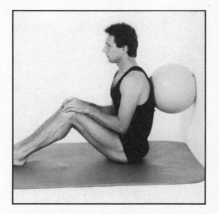
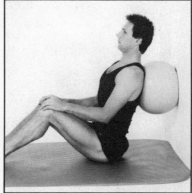

<u>*Level 2:*</u>
Sitting, pull back, using a cable as resistance in a "tug-of-war."

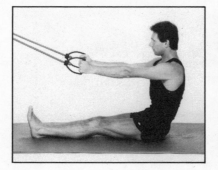
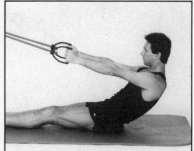

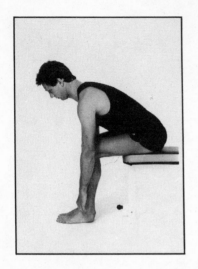
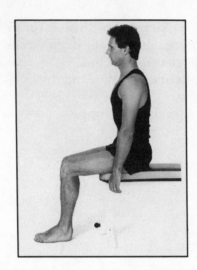

Level 3:
Sit with your feet shoulder width apart, bending over. Straighten up.

Level 4:
a. Same as level 3, with weight held at chest.

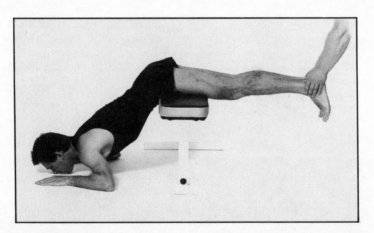

b. Lie stomach-down across a bench with your feet anchored and your upper body over the edge. Arch up to a horizontal position, using your arms for support.

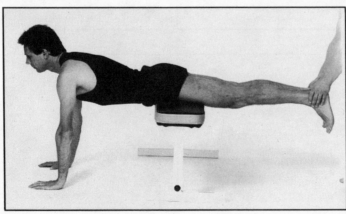

Level 5:

Same as level 4b, with hands held behind your head or on your chest.

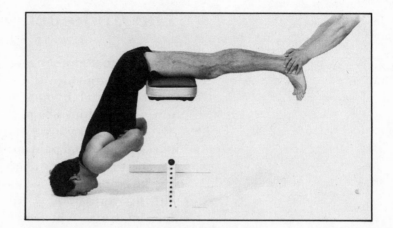

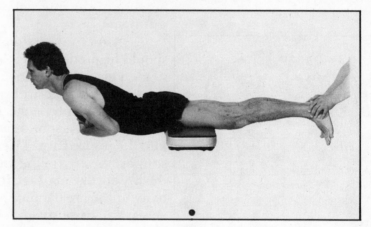

The Abdomen

Making the abdomen stronger and healthier helps to provide support for the lower back and helps you return to normal if you have had abdominal surgery or an abdominal muscle pull.

Ron is a young man who for five years experienced abdominal pain and weakness from his stomach down into his groin due to a torn muscle. It got so bad that he couldn't play an easy game of tennis or wrestle with his young son. I treated him with exercise and deep massage, which here requires extreme caution because of the internal organs located just under the soft tissue.

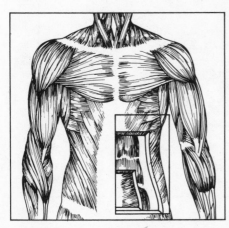

After any abdominal or chest surgery, you should begin deep-breathing exercises as soon as possible. This can be done as soon after the surgery as physically possible with medical clearance. Begin by breathing deeply while supporting the tender area with a pillow. As soon as possible, try isolated breathing into the injured area by exhaling, using your hands to support the area of the incision. Adding pressure from the inside, like massage from the outside, increases activity in the area and improves blood circulation, prevents scar tissue from forming and causing atrophy, and helps the area return to normal function. Without the breathing exercises, you become more susceptible to respiratory problems.

To start, you should begin with the level 1 abdominal exercises once you have been given medical clearance to do so. While in your hospital bed you can begin to lean forward gently while holding on to the area of the incision or do simple stretching exercises, such as lifting a yardstick directly overhead from your thighs.

Massage

Not recommended except by tissue-restorative massage specialist.

Exercises

Level 1:
Backlying in a semi-reclined position, sitting or standing, lean forward while pulling on a cable.

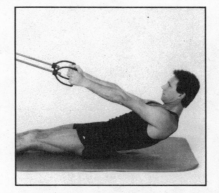 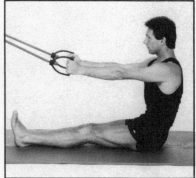

Level 2:
Lie on your side and curl your upper body to your legs and vice versa.

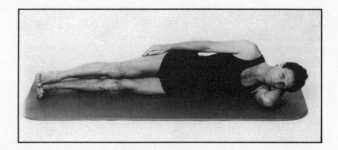

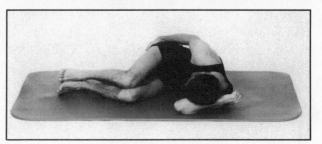

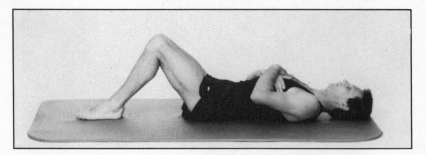

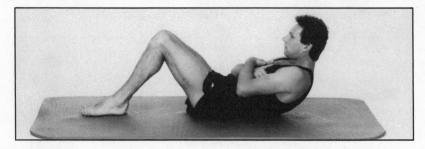

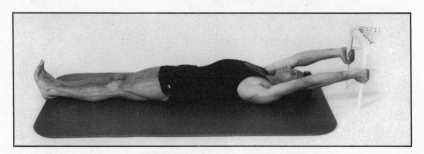

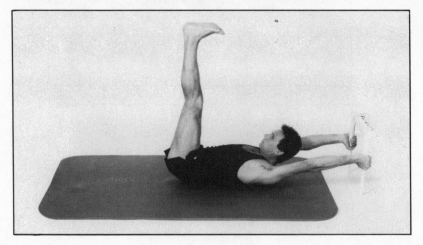

Level 3:

a. Lie on your back with your feet on the floor and knees bent. Tuck your chin to your chest, lifting your upper body until your shoulder blades clear the ground. Continue until you can lift your middle back off the ground. Vary the position of your arms by putting them at your side, crossing them over your chest, and placing your hands at the sides of your head.

b. Lie on your back with your hands anchored above and behind you. Raising your head up and pressing your lower back against the floor, lift one leg at a time and then both legs at once.

c. Sideovers—Lying on your back with knees flexed at 90 degrees at your side, lift your knees up until your buttocks are flat against the floor.

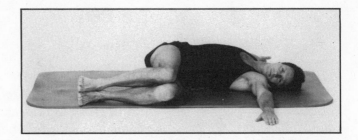

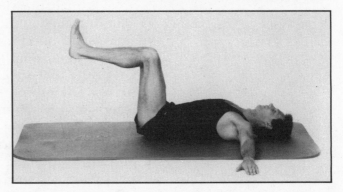

Level 4:
   a. Same as level 3b, on an incline board.
   b. Same as level 3c (sideovers) with legs straight.

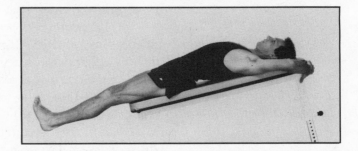

Level 5:
   a. Same as level 4a, adding resistance with ankle weights.

   b. Same as level 4b, adding resistance with ankle weights.

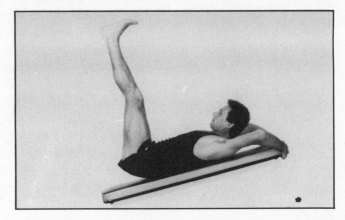

The Hip

The hip is a ball-and-socket joint like the shoulder, but due to the stability needed for upright position, it is not nearly as mobile. The hip joint has more muscles crossing over it than any other joint in the body.

The main muscle in the hip area is the iliopsoas, which is attached to the spine and crosses in front of the pelvis to connect to the hipbone. A group of muscles in the inner thigh called the adductors draw the legs together and stabilize them when we walk. The rectus femoris, one of the four muscles in the front of the thigh, attaches to the pelvis and crosses the knee. The hamstrings extend from under the buttocks to behind the knee in the back of the thigh and are involved in propulsive movements (such as jumping, leaping, and hopping), walking, running, climbing, and standing. On the outside, the gluteal muscles, the iliotibial band, and the deep rotators are the key muscles.

The major problems I have run into involve the soft tissue around the hip, specifically within the areas of the gluteal fascia, the iliotibial band, and the rectus femoris, which runs across the front of the thigh and is the longest of the muscles comprising the quadriceps. These are all very vulnerable areas, as they absorb a great deal of shock from the lower body. Even dancers, whose legs tend to be long and lean, are very susceptible to rectus femoris tendonitis, which involves the muscle soreness in the muscle that helps lift the leg. Many runners tend to have problems with the iliotibial band and the hamstrings in the back of the thigh.

Hamstring strains can occur from the bottom of the pelvis to below the back of the knee. Pain in the back of the thigh usually indicates a muscle tear, while pain in the buttocks or behind the knee tends to mean tendon problems. The injuries may be very deep and require deep manual evaluation to find the N-bodies. Hamstring injuries to the muscles or tendons respond best to deep massage and exercise.

Sandra, a teacher in her late forties, was told that her hip pain was caused by osteoarthritis. Four different specialists suggested that she rest, stop playing tennis, walk with crutches or a cane, and take anti-inflammatory medication. As a result of her inactivity, the range of motion in her hip became limited. She came to me complaining of pain in the right hip area, outside of the thigh down to her knee, and in the upper right side of her pelvis. I found N-body formation and tightened fascia around her hip and tightness in her iliotibial band down to her knees. The treatment was massage and exercise.

Carol, a ballet dancer, came to me with complaints of pain in her hip and the upper front of her thigh. She was told that because she danced ballet, she already had the beginnings of arthritis, a problem that would grow worse as she aged. Again, my evaluation discovered N-bodies on the tendon of the rectus femoris muscles on the front of the thigh. This was a result of the stress of flexing her straight leg when she assumed the turned-out position characteristic of dance. Deep massage and strengthening exercises corrected the problem.

I first met Lindy when she was six years old. This little girl suffered from Legg-Perthes, a disease that affects the hips (and is not unlike the osteochondritis dissecans I suffered from as a child). By the time her parents brought her to my office, she had already spent six months in casts that extended on both sides from her hips to her chest and was understandably shy of anyone touching her. The casts had caused complicated back problems and left her without any range of motion on the left side of her hip.

The specialist had told her mother not to worry, that the situation did not require any physical therapy and would heal by itself. However, if Lindy had stayed inactive for much longer, she would have been crippled. Lindy and I began therapy. At first she resisted, crying and screaming. Progress was slow.

The story, however, had a happy ending. After two years of treatment, three times a week, she has regained full range of motion and normal muscle power. At her last physical examination, her specialist turned to his intern and said, "You see, these problems always correct themselves in children." (Tell me about it!)

Other common soft-tissue injuries to the hip and thigh area include hip pointer (a ripping away of the tendons attached to the iliac crest), trochanteric bursitis (an inflammation of the bursa sac that is just above the thighbone), and what is often referred to as a charley horse, which also affects the arms (a bruise that "knots up" the skin).

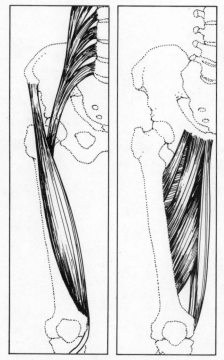

Circle 1 - (front) Common injuries: quadricep strains, rectus femoris tendonitis, iliopoas bursitis, sartorial avulsion. Exercise: hip flexion

Circle 2 - (inside) Common injury: groin pulls. Exercises: hip adduction, flexion, extension

Circle 3 - (outside) Common injuries: iliotibial band problems, trochanteric bursitis, hip pointer. Exercises: hip abduction, flexion, extension

Circle 4 - (back) Common injuries: hamstring pulls, sciatic nerve impingement. Exercises: hip extension and rotation

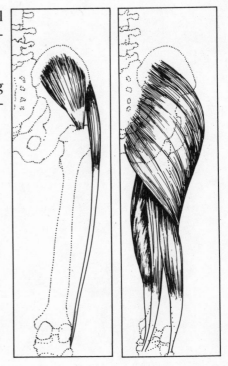

Massage

Front of Thigh (quadriceps)

1. Lie on your back with both legs out straight and a pillow under your knees for comfort.

2. Spread cream from just below the knee to the groin.

3. Start with a superficial effleurage using both hands massaging upward from the knee to the groin.

4. Now do a deeper effleurage over the same area using the heels of both hands. You can alternate this with the first three fingers of both hands.

5. Begin petrissage. Work up from the knee to the groin.

6. Now do a friction massage using the thumbs of both hands to make deep circles working upward from the knee to the groin.

7. Follow friction with a deep horizontal wringing motion. With both hands placed horizontally across the thigh just above the knee, massage upward in a wringing motion.

8. Repeat deep effleurage with the heels of both hands from the knee up to the groin.

9. End with a superficial effleurage over the same area.

Back of Thigh (hamstrings)

1. Lie on your stomach with your lower legs supported on a pillow for comfort.

2. Follow the massage steps for the front of the thigh.

Side of Thigh (iliotibial band)

1. Lie on your side with your top leg bent on a pillow for comfort.

2. Follow the massage steps for the front of the thigh.

Exercises

Hip Flexion

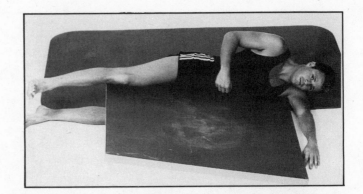

Level 1:
Lie on your side with your leg (either bent or straight) on the highest portion of a decline board. Move your leg toward your head.

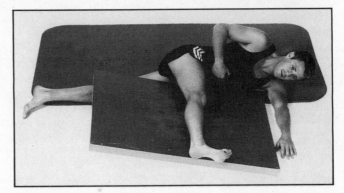

Level 2:
Same as level 1, with leg on level surface.

Level 3:
Sitting or standing, bend your knee up toward your chest.

Level 4:
Same as level 3, adding resistance with a weight on your ankle.

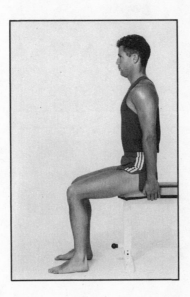
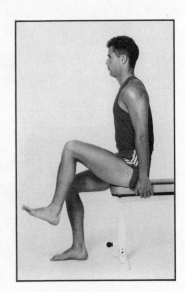

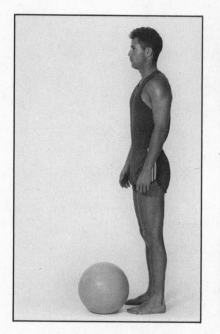

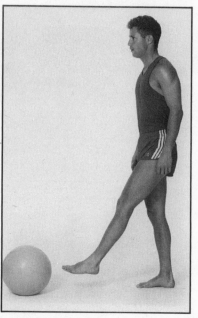

Level 5:

Standing, kick a ball forward, keeping your leg straight.

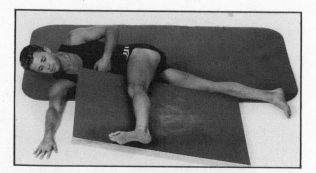

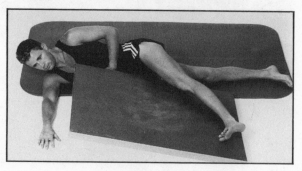

Hip Extension

Level 1:

Lie on your side with your leg (either bent or straight) on the highest portion of a decline board. Move your leg down the decline away from your head.

Level 2:

Same as level 1, with leg on level surface.

Level 3:
Lying prone over a bench with your feet touching the ground and your legs straight, lift each leg separately.

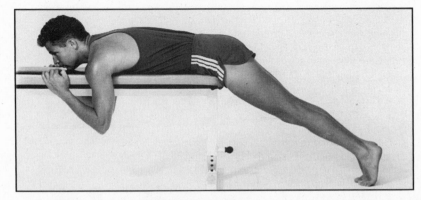

Level 4:
Same as level 3, adding resistance with a weight on each ankle.

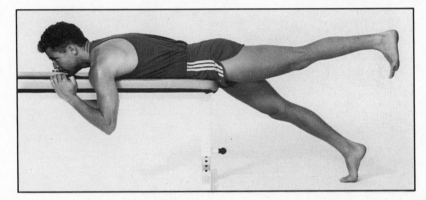

Level 5:
a. Split squat, starting with the front knee bent, move to standing.

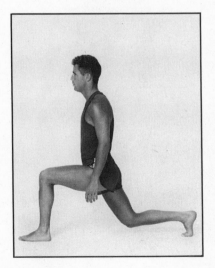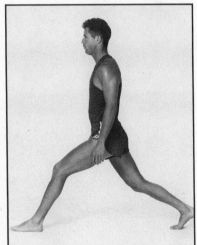

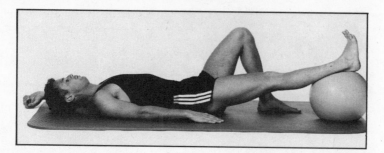

b. Lie on your back with a wedge or ball under your ankle and your leg straight. Push down on the wedge or ball to lift your hips off the floor.

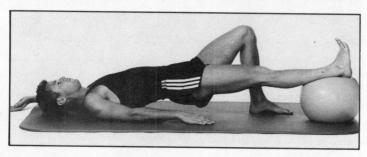

Hip Abduction

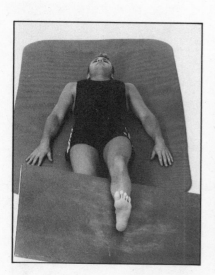

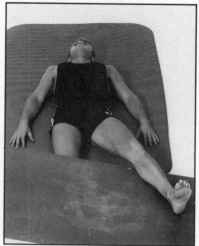

Level 1:
Lie on your back with your leg on a board tilting away from your body. Keeping your leg straight, slide it down the board to the side.

Level 2:
Same as level 1, with your leg on level ground.

Level 3:
Lie on your side and lift your top leg toward the ceiling.

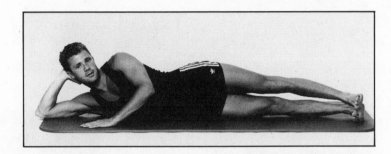

Level 4:
Same as level 3, adding resistance with a weight on your ankle.

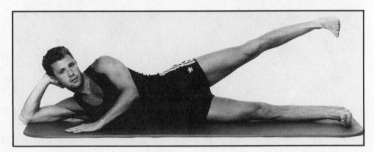

Level 5:
Standing, lift your leg out to the side against a ball weight or rubber cable, keeping your leg straight.

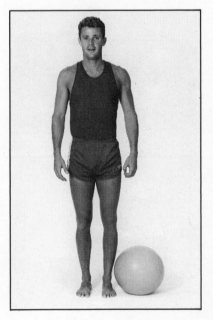 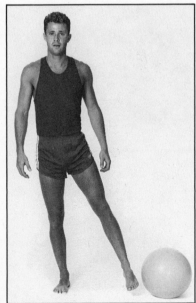

Hip Adduction

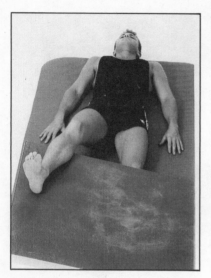
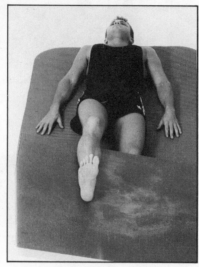

Level 1:
    Lie on your back with your leg on a board tilting in toward your body. Keeping the leg straight, slide it down the board toward the other leg.

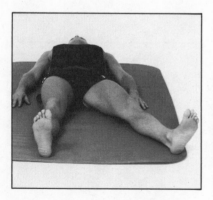
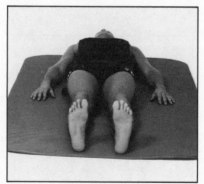

Level 2:
    Lie on your back with your legs straight and spread apart. Keep one leg stationary and move the other leg toward it.

Level 3:

Sidelying with your top leg on a chair or bench, lift your injured leg up toward the top one.

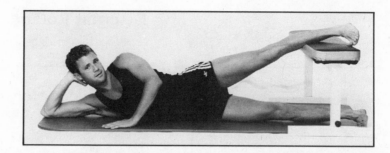

Level 4:

Same as level 3, adding resistance on the bottom leg.

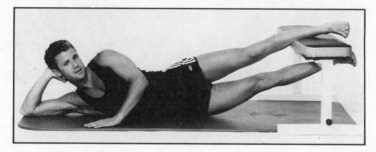

Level 5:

Standing with foot on injured side forward and the other diagonally back, squat to the side over your forward foot and return to the starting position.

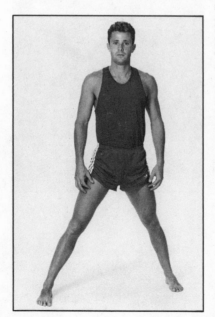
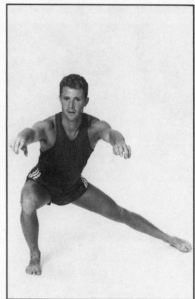

Hip External Rotation

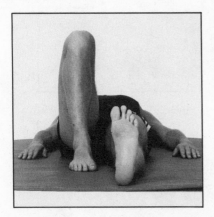
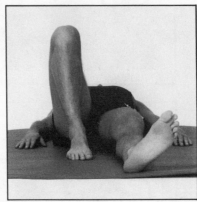

Level 1:

Lie on your back with one leg bent and the other straight. Rotate your straight leg to the side.

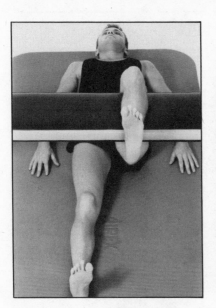
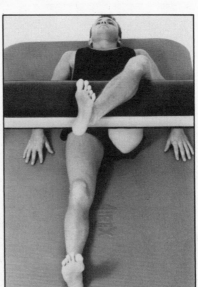

Level 2:

Lie on your back with one leg bent over a bench. Move your foot to the inside, keeping the knee stationary.

Level 3:

Sit on a bench with your lower legs hanging freely. Move the lower leg toward the other leg.

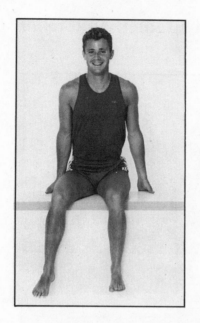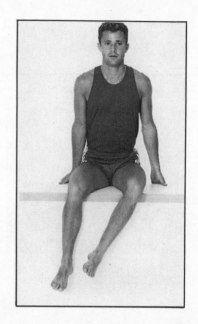

Level 4:

Same as level 3, adding resistance with a rubber cable.

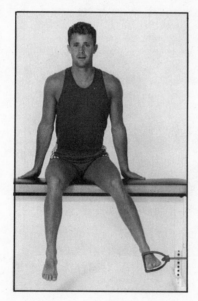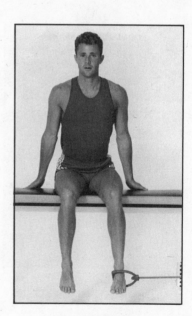

Hip Internal Rotation

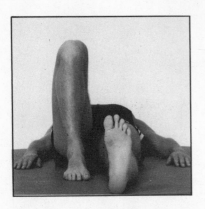 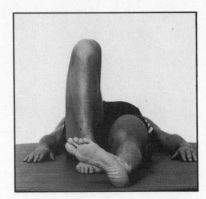

Level 1:
Lie on your back with one leg bent and the other straight. Rotate the straight leg inward.

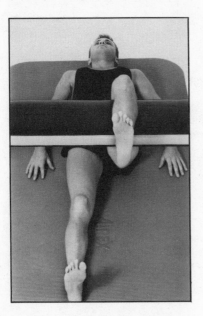 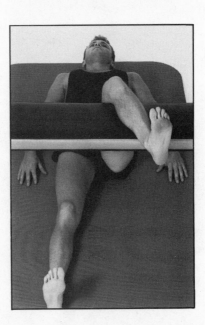

Level 2:
Lie on your back with one leg bent over a bench. Move the foot outward, keeping knee stationary.

Level 3:
Sit on a bench with your lower legs hanging freely. Move the lower leg out away from the other leg.

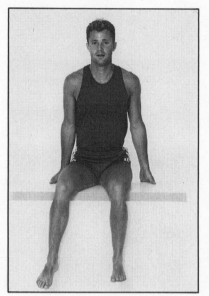 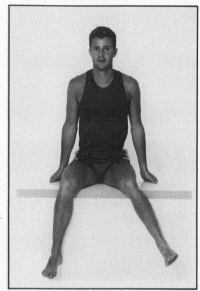

Level 4:
Same as level 3, adding resistance with a rubber cable.

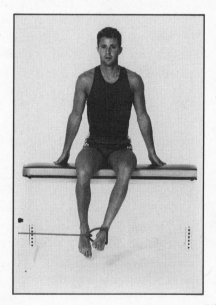 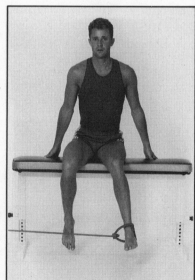

The Knee

The knee is the joint where the long bone of the upper leg joins with the bones of the lower leg. The leg bones are the longest bones in the body, yet it is this length that is a contributing factor in many knee injuries.

Held together by a series of ligaments, the knees' strongest and most vulnerable ligaments are on the inside—the medial collateral—and the outside—the lateral collateral. The ligaments that cross each other inside are the cruciate. Also on the outside of the knee is the iliotibial band. The kneecap is held in place by the retinaculum and patellar tendon.

Bursas, tendons, and ligaments comprise the top and bottom of the kneecaps. Below the kneecap and toward the inside of the shinbone is an area where three tendons meet with a bursa underneath. Shaped like a goose's foot, this area's Latin name is *pes anserinus*. This is a common area for tendonitis and bursitis. Chondromalacia, a softening and thinning of the underside cartilage of the kneecap, can also produce pain.

Another pain-producing condition is water on the knee, an irritation of the lining of the knee joint caused by a ligament or cartilage injury. The shock of the injury causes parts of the knee to produce excess fluid in the area, which puts pressure on the joint. In most cases, the fluid disappears with the healing of the primary injury.

I can't begin to count the number of times I have treated ligaments, tendons, and other soft-tissue injuries in the knee that were mistaken for cartilage tears. These soft tissues can almost always be treated successfully by my methods. True cartilage damage and complete ligament tears, however, require surgery.

Dawn, a soccer player at the college where I began my private practice, twisted her knee during a game. Her knee spasmed and swelled to such a degree that she could not straighten it. X rays were negative, but she was told by the specialists that she had torn cartilage, which needed to be removed immediately—no conservative methods, no physical therapy, just immediate surgery.

Dawn remembered that I had helped the same knee, for a different injury, the year before. This time, my hands-on evaluation revealed a second-degree tear of her medial collateral ligament, as well as second-degree strains of her hamstring tendon and calf tendons in the back of her knee. Ten weeks of deep massage and exercise left her stronger than ever. The slight bend in her knee remained, which required long-term extensive treatments to correct.

When she returned to the specialist for a release to play again, she was told that the slight bend in her knee was a result of cartilage getting stuck in the joint and that it could be cured only with surgery. She underwent arthroscopic surgery, and no cartilage damage was found.

Although many specialists believe that arthroscopic surgery is not a really involved procedure, this is hardly an excuse for having it when any knee problem presents itself. Surgery should always be the final option. All conservative methods should be exhausted before any part of the body undergoes surgery.

Frank, a psychologist, twisted his knee while pushing his young daughter on the swings. X ray results were negative, but his orthopedist scheduled him the following week for surgery to repair a torn cartilage. Through a manual evaluation of the area, I concluded that the problem was the result of damage in the soft tissue surrounding his kneecap. I told him what I tell all people I work with—treat conservatively first. Strengthen and make the area healthier through massage and exercise before you consider anything else. Frank's treatment was successful.

Becky came to me complaining of excruciating pain that occurred after two knee surgeries. The first surgery was to remove a piece of torn cartilage. The pain, however, remained. The second surgeon reoperated to "clean out" the scar tissue in her knee. Again, there was no improvement. Six months later, his response was that the problem was not in her knee but in her head. Other specialists concurred. She started to wonder if maybe they were right.

In the meantime, the pain was so intense that she was forced to quit her job. One surgeon had a final solution: fuse the knee, which would leave it permanently stiffened and unable to bend (which is not quite what an active twenty-six-year-old wants to hear). I worked on her knee for several months—again using massage and exercise—before I was able to begin breaking down what I thought was scar tissue on the nerve endings that had formed as a result of the surgeries and caused her such agony. It took about nine months before Becky's pain began to subside. She is still coming to see me regularly, and her condition continues to improve.

Mary was also planning to undergo surgery for a cartilage tear. She had injured her knee while skiing down the beginner's hill. Her actual injury was pes anserinus bursitis tendonitis, or goose-foot bursitis, which is an irritation in the bursa sac that lies under the tendons on the inner side of the knee. This condition is the second most common type of bursitis in the knee, next to prepatella bursitis, or "housemaid's knee" (historically this was considered an occupational hazard for those who made their living scrubbing floors, supporting themselves on their knees and elbows). Both of these injuries respond well to massage and exercise. Mary did fine without the surgery.

Roger, a triathlete, had severe pain on the outside of his knee from an iliotibial-band inflammation that put pressure on the nerves that shot into his knee. He was improving from my therapy but wanted to speed up his recovery time so that he could return to his training. He underwent arthroscopic surgery for what his surgeon diagnosed as synovial plica (an extra ridge of scar tissue that folds over on itself and begins to rub against the surface of the joint). Instead of getting back on his feet more quickly after the surgery, he was sidelined for weeks until he continued the same restorative program he had been too impatient to follow.

Tom, a high school wrestler, was told by his physician that he had a torn cartilage in his knee. Rest was recommended. It turned out that he had a simple hamstring tear, easily treated with massage and exercise. Unfortunately, Tom ended up wearing a knee brace and a shoe orthotic insert over the next four months. No physical therapy was prescribed, and as a result, he did not improve. He missed the entire season, which was a shame because once I got my hands on him, the injury was healed after ten sessions.

Finally, Rick Carey, the gold-medal-winning swimmer in the 1984 Olympics, hurt his knee during training, then reinjured it while stretching. He was told that he had dislocated his kneecap and that it would take twelve weeks to heal. This would have kept him out of the water for a good part of the season. Whether or not it involved dislocation, Rick's problem was a soft-tissue strain. I immediately put him on a restorative program of two deep massages a day and exercise that had him back in the pool within two weeks at full function.

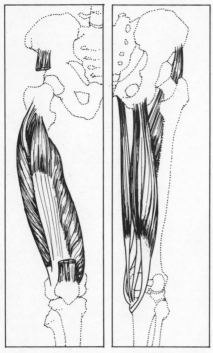

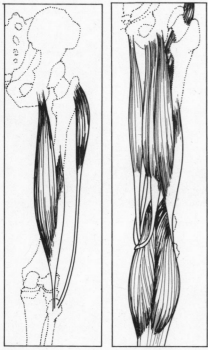

Circle 1 - (front) Common injuries: quadricep strains and tendonitis, chondromalacia, patellar tendonitis and bursitis, medial and lateral retinaculum tears, ligament injuries of the area. Exercises: hip flexion, knee extension

Circle 2 - (inside) Common injuries: Pes anserinus bursitis, medial collateral ligament tears, hamstring tendonitis, sartorius muscle/tendon strain. Exercise: knee extension with foot inversion

Circle 3 - (outside) Common injuries: lateral hamstring tendonitis, iliotibial strain, lateral collateral ligament tear. Exercises: hip abduction, knee extension and flexion with foot everted

Circle 4 - (back) Common injuries: hamstring muscle tear, hyperextended knee, calf muscle strains, popliteal muscle tear. Exercises: hip extension, knee flexion

Massage:

1. Sit with your knee bent to a 45-degree angle. For comfort, support the knee on a pillow.

2. Spread cream from the midshin to the midthigh area.

3. Start with a superficial effleurage using both hands, massaging upward from the midshin to the midthigh.

4. Now do a deeper effleurage using the first three fingers of both hands, outlining the kneecap.

5. Begin friction using the thumbs of both hands to make small circles along both sides of the shinbone, moving upward to outline the kneecap.

6. Continue friction using the thumb and first two fingers of both hands to grab and pull tissue just below the knee and along the kneecap.

7. Follow friction with a deep effleurage.

8. Now repeat steps 5 and 6.

9. Follow with a deep effleurage again.

10. End with a superficial effleurage.

Knee Extension

<u>Level 1:</u>

Lie on your back and place a towel under your knee. Push the back of the knee into the towel.

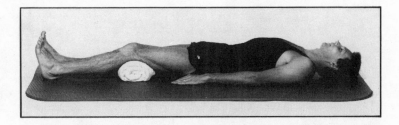

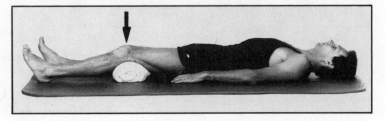

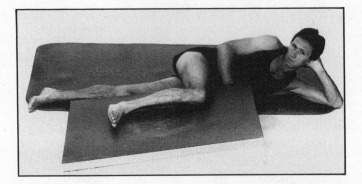

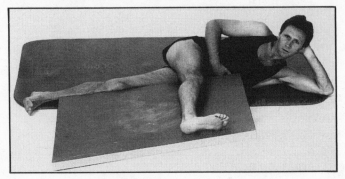

Level 2:

Lie on your side with your leg out straight on the peak of a decline board. Bend your knee, moving the leg down the board.

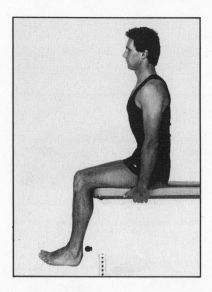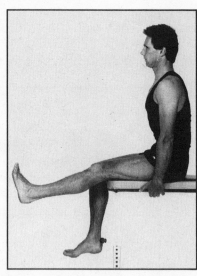

Level 3:

Sit on the edge of a table with your legs hanging freely. Lift your lower leg toward the ceiling and hold for two seconds. Slowly return to the starting position and repeat. Turn your foot in to work the inner knee area or out to work the outer knee.

Level 4:

Same as level 3, adding resistance.

Level 5:

a. Perform a split squat holding two chairs for support. If your knee won't bend to 90 degrees, repeat the exercise, progressively working your way down and back up again. Once you've achieved balance, perform a split squat:
(1) Holding one chair for support
(2) With no support
(3) With weights in hand

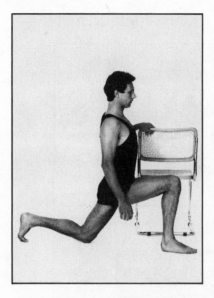
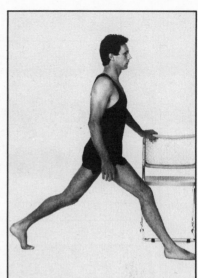

b. With your back against the wall, slide down so that your thighs are perpendicular to the floor. Hold for one minute, then return to the starting position.

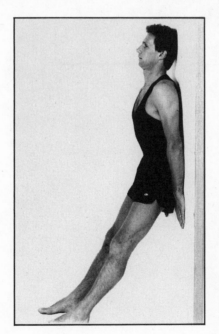
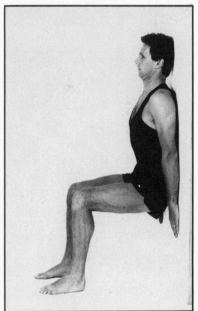

Knee Flexion:

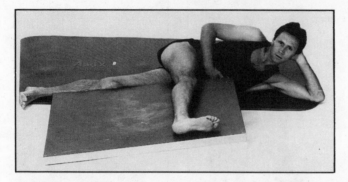

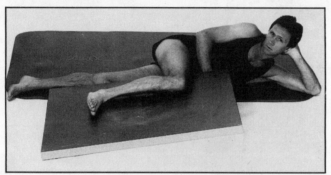

Level 1:
  Lie on your side with your bent leg resting on the peak of a decline board. Move your leg down the board.

Level 2:
  Same as level 1, keeping the board level.

<u>*Level 3:*</u>

Lie stomach-down
on bench with your
knee supported and
slightly bent. Bend
your knee to 90
degrees.

<u>*Level 4*</u>:

Same as level 3, add-
ing resistance with a
weight on the ankle.

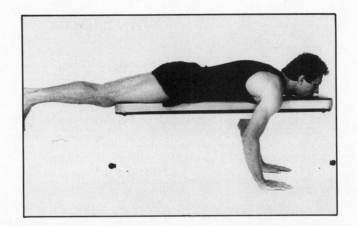

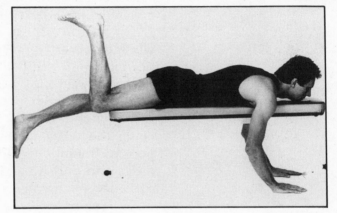

The Elbow

The elbow is the joint that connects the bone in the upper arm to the bones in the lower arm (forearm). Problems bending or straightening the elbow will show an inflammation in the elbow joint itself. Most elbow injuries, however, are not found in the joint itself, but in the ligaments and tendons of the muscles that surround and control the elbow, wrist, and hand movements. The most common elbow injuries are tennis elbow (lateral epicondylitis), where you feel pain outside the elbow, and pitcher's or golfer's elbow (medial epicondylitis), where the pain is felt on the inside.

Sharon came to me after suffering from tennis elbow for about two years. She had been forced to stop playing tennis and had gone the typical route, trying virtually everything—cortisone shots, pills, physical therapy (although not my methods), and acupuncture—without success. Her problem, which ended up being the result of poor posture and consequenty, poor techniques, resulted in N-bodies on her outside lower-arm muscles and tendons. After being treated correctly, she has never had the problem again.

Tennis elbow is not restricted to people like Sharon who play tennis with poor posture, less-than-ideal form, or improper equipment. People who knit, work on assembly lines, or give massages for hours at a time, as I do, are just as prone to this injury. Basically anyone who does continuous and shocking work with his arm is a candidate for tennis elbow. There are usually one or more factors involved: overuse, poor technique, bad posture in the shoulders, poor warm-up, and muscle weakness in the forearm. My experiences with this injury have shown that it takes the longest time to heal of any soft-tissue injury.

Jack had more advanced tennis elbow which resulted in a painful pressure on the nerve between his forearm muscles. This, in turn, caused a general tightness all over his arm and a permanent limitation of motion at the elbow. A top squash player, Jack was also tight in his shoulders, upper back, and lower back. His condition forced him to play more with his arm, rather than his whole body, creating an added stress that further aggravated the situation. We got rid of the pain in his elbow, but Jack also had to begin learning how to stretch out his entire upper body to prevent the problem that had caused the elbow injury in the first place.

Pitcher's or golfer's elbow can happen to pot scrubbers as well as to major-league hurlers and members of the professional golfers' tour. The injury is the result of a strain on the inside of the elbow. As with tennis elbow, it is usually caused by repetitive overuse of the muscle, which in this case is the attachment at the inner knob of the elbow (medial epicondyle). In a severe case, pain may travel from the elbow down to the wrist. It is nearly as common, and just as painful, as tennis elbow.

These inside and outside areas of the elbow overlap each other so much that it is often hard to isolate the injury without good manual evaluation skills. Joe, a weight lifter, was treated for six months by other specialists for golfer's elbow without feeling any better. He was not improving because the problem was actually higher up his arm, in his tricep tendons, as the discovery of small N-bodies in the area indicated.

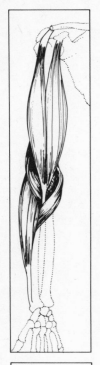
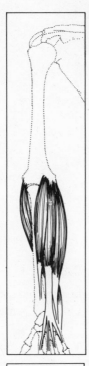

Circle 1 - (front) Common injuries: bicep tendonitis, brachialis coracobrachialis, strains of the supinator and pronator muscles. Exercises: elbow flexion, pronation, and supination

Circle 2 - (inside) Common injuries: pitcher's or golfer's elbow, ulnar neuritis. Exercises: elbow flexion, wrist flexion

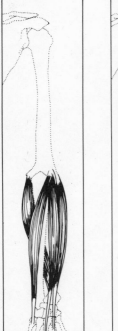
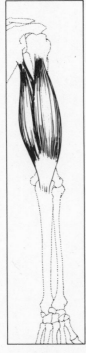

Circle 3 - (outside) Common injuries: tennis elbow, wrist-extension muscle tendon strains, brachioradialis. Exercises: elbow flexion, wrist extension

Circle 4 - (back) Common injuries: tricep tendonitis, tricep bursitis. Exercise: elbow extension

Massage

Front of Elbow

1. Sit with arm supported on a table and elbow slightly bent over a pillow for comfort.

2. Spread cream from the wrist up to the upper arm, covering both sides of the arm.

3. Start with superficial effleurage, using one or two hands, massaging from the wrist to the upper arm.

4. Now do a deeper effleurage using the heel of one or both of your hands over the same area. You can alternate this with the first three fingers of one or both of your hands.

5. Begin petrissage, using the thumb and first two fingers of both hands to grab and pull the tissue. Concentrate on the area around the elbow crease.

6. Now do a friction massage, using both thumbs in small, deep circles, covering the area from the mid-forearm to the mid-upper arm.

7. Follow friction with a wringing massage. Place both hands horizontally on the forearm, massaging up to the upper arm in a wringing motion.

8. Repeat petrissage.

9. Repeat deep effleurage.

10. End with superficial effleurage.

Back of Elbow

1. Lie on your stomach with your arm at your side in a relaxed position.

2. Follow the same massage steps as for the front of the elbow.

Exercises

Elbow Flexion

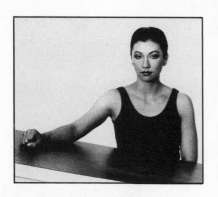
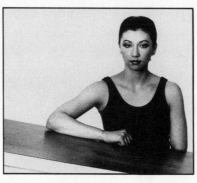

Level 1:
Sit with your hand on the peak of a wedge, with elbow bent. Slide your hand down wedge.

Level 2:
Same as level 1, with hand on level surface.

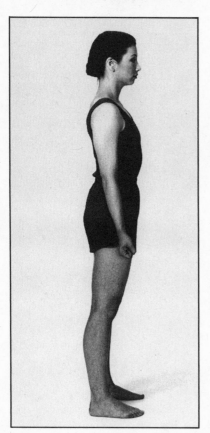
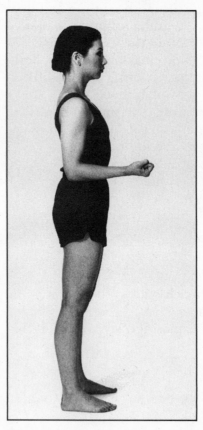

Level 3:
a. Stand with your arm at your side. Bend your elbow repeatedly with your palm facing up.

b. Sit with out-stretched arm supported on a table. Beginning with your palm facing upward, bend your elbow to 90 degrees.

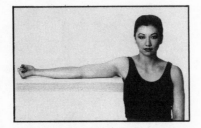
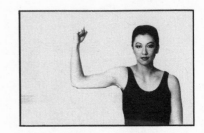

c. Standing with your arm straight at your side, bend your elbow to 90 degrees with your palm facing downward.

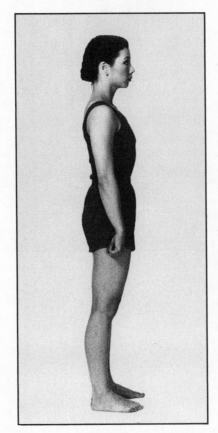
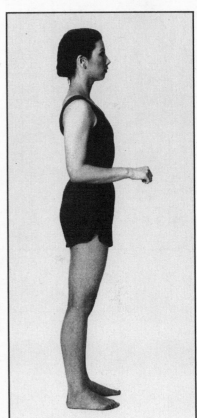

Level 4:
Same as levels 3a, 3b, and 3c, adding resistance by adding a weight.

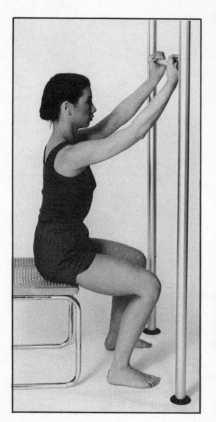
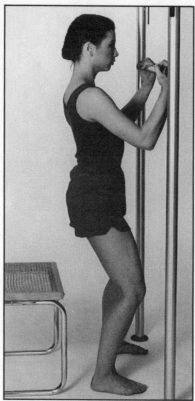

Level 5:

   a. Gripping a bar with palms toward you, do chin-ups from a sitting position. Pull up to a standing position until your elbows are flexed.

b. Either standing or sitting, do curls using dumbbells as resistance.

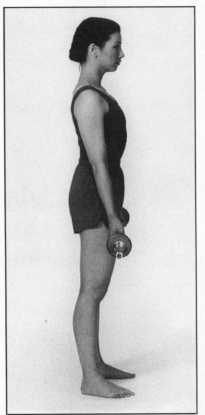 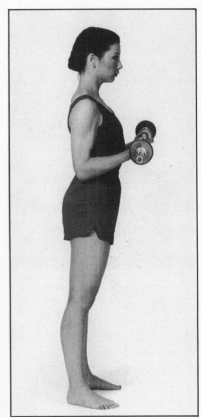

Elbow Extension

Level 1:

Lie on your side with bent arm on the peak of a board declined away from your head. Straighten your arm, moving the forearm down the board.

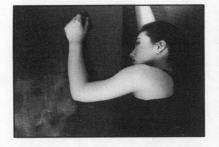 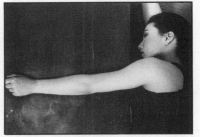

Level 2:

Same as level 1, keeping the board level.

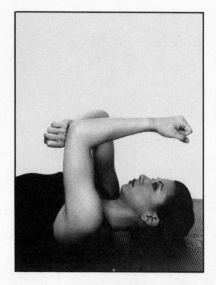 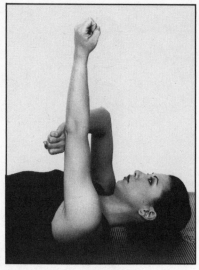

Level 3:

Lie on your back with your arm raised to a 90-degree angle and your elbow bent. Straighten your arm upward.

Level 4:

Same as level 3, adding resistance on your wrist.

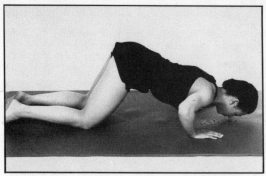

Level 5:

a. On your hands and knees, do push-ups, keeping your chest out and your stomach in. To make this exercise more demanding, either extend your legs or raise your feet up on a bench.

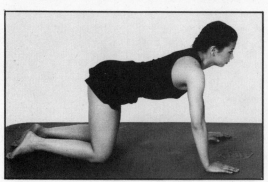

b. Squat on the floor between two boxes. With each hand on a box, push yourself up. As you repeat this exercise, extend your legs out until you can do this from a sitting position.

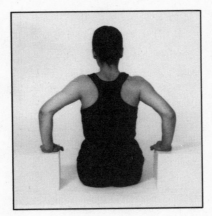 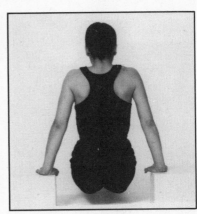

Elbow Pronation/Supination

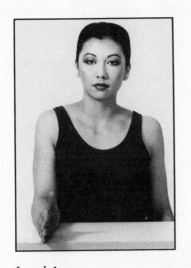 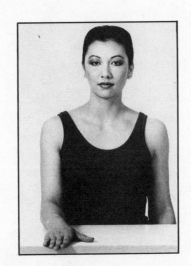 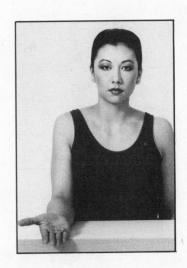

Level 1:

Lie on your back with your hand open and your thumb pointing up. Turn your palm down (pronation), then up (supination).

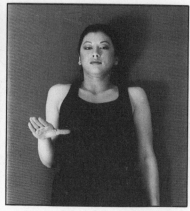
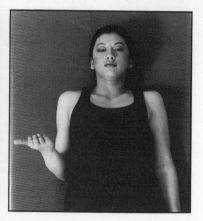
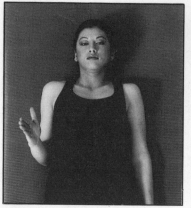

Level 2:
Lie on your back with upper arm against your body and elbow bent 90 degrees. Rotate your hand so that your thumb moves toward your body (pronation) and away from your body (supination).

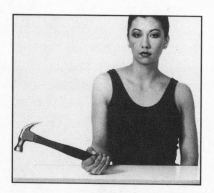
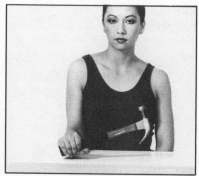

Level 3:
Sit with your elbow bent to 90 degrees, fist closed and thumb up. Turn your hand palm down (pronation) and then palm up (supination). (Refer to photo for level 4, without hammer.)

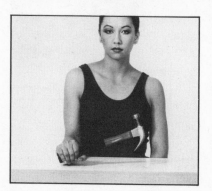
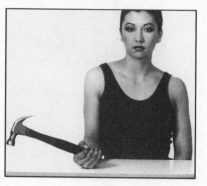

Level 4:
Same as level 3, holding a weight, such as a hammer, in your hand.

Level 5:

Sit with your elbow
bent to 90 degrees.
Hold a short stick with
a weight attached on
the end with a rope.
Turn the stick as if
turning a screwdriver,
first to the left, then to
the starting position,
then to the right.

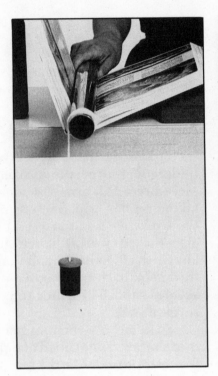 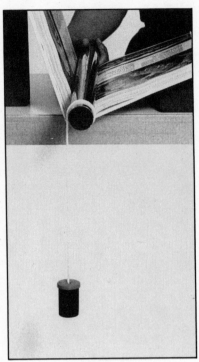

The Wrist

Injuries to the wrist are usually in the tendons, the ligaments or the bones, the first two of which are best treated by deep massage and exercise. The most common injury, a sprain, is an injury to the ligaments in the wrist.

I also see patients who have wrist problems after undergoing surgery for broken bones. Fran, for example, wore a full arm cast for six to eight weeks after falling on her arm. She was not encouraged to move the arm while it was in a cast or for a number of weeks after the cast was off. Later, she found herself without any wrist, elbow or shoulder mobility. She needed to be treated for each area, both by itself and as a unit. It took several months for her to return to a healthy pre-surgical state.

Jamie, a woman in her thirties who makes her own clothes, complained of tightness around her wrists which appeared to be the result of too much knitting. A specialist diagnosed her problem as carpal tunnel syndrome, where tight tissues and N-bodies around the wrist cause pressure on the nerves to the hand. With this injury, pain in the wrist may extend up the forearm or down into the hand, with tingling or numbness in the fingertips.

Massage and exercise take care of the injury as effectively as and more naturally than other methods. Jamie's pain was relieved after a dozen or so sessions, and she returned to her knitting.

Circle 1 - (front) Common injuries: carpal tunnel syndrome, trigger finger, muscle strain. Exercise: wrist flexion.

Circle 2 - (inside) Common injuries: deQuervain's disease, ligament and tendon strains. Exercise: ulnar deviation.

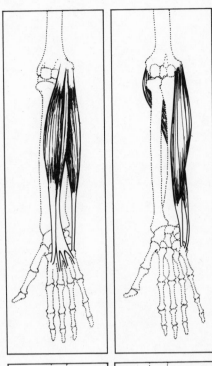

Circle 3 - (outside) Common injuries: tenosynovitis, ligament and tendon strains. Exercise: radial deviation.

Circle 4 - (back) Common injuries: muscle sprains, tenosynovitis, referred pain from nerve compression (see neck). Exercise: wrist extension.

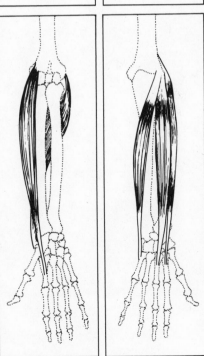

Massage

1. Sit with the forearm supported on a table.

2. Spread cream from the tips of the fingers to the middle of the forearm.

3. Start with superficial effleurage. Use your whole hand, massaging from the tips of the fingers to the middle of the forearm.

4. Now do a deeper effleurage, using your whole hand or the first three fingers of your hand.

5. Continue with a deep effleurage, using both thumbs to massage each finger separately with deep, longitudinal strokes on the top, bottom, and sides of the fingers, massaging up to the hand and wrist.

6. Begin a friction massage using both thumbs to massage in small circles, working each finger separately and moving up to the hand and wrist. Also massage the soft tissue between each finger.

7. Now massage the thumbs of the patient with a deep effleurage, using both the thumbs of the healer in a deep, longitudinal stroke on the top, bottom, and sides up to the wrist.

8. Now do friction massage to the thumbs using both of the healer's thumbs to make small circles from the tip up to the wrist. Also massage the soft tissue between the thumb and fingers.

9. Follow the friction massage with deep effleurage to the whole hand.

10. End with superficial effleurage to the whole hand.

Exercises

Wrist Extension

Level 1:
Sit with your fore-arm supported over a bench, palm facing up, and elbow either bent or straight. Let your wrist drop back.

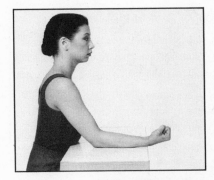 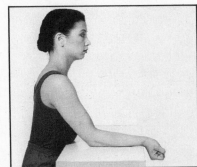

Level 2:
Sit with your fore-arm supported, thumb up, and wrist straight. Bend your wrist back.

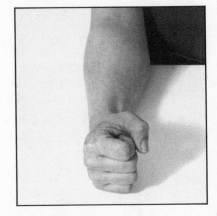 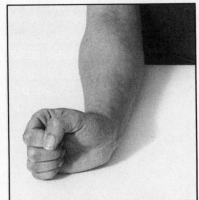

Level 3:
Sit with your fore-arm supported and palm facing down. Bend your wrist back.

Level 4:
Same as level 3, add-ing resistance by hold-ing on to a bar.

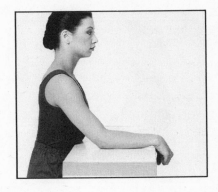 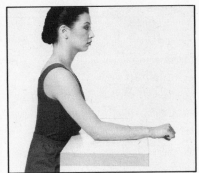

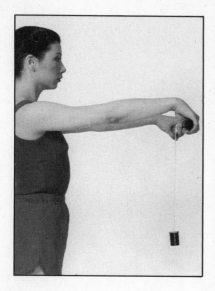 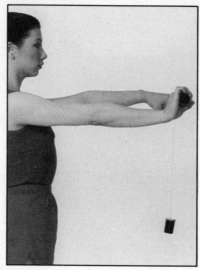

Level 5:
    With elbows either bent or straight, hold a bar with both hands, palms facing down. Alternating hands, roll the bar toward you.

Wrist Flexion

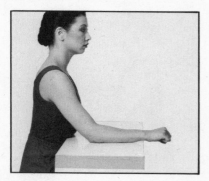 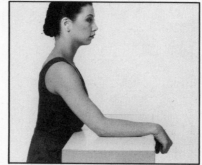

Level 1:
    Sit with your forearm supported over a bench, palm facing down and elbow either bent or straight. Move your wrist downward.

Level 2:

Sit with your fore-arm supported, thumb up and wrist straight. Bend your wrist forward.

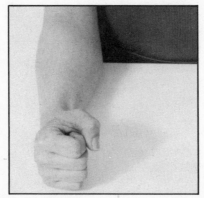

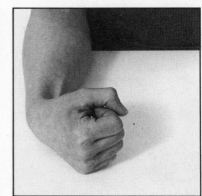

Level 3:

Sit with your fore-arm supported and palm facing up. Bend your wrist up.

Level 4:

Same as level 3, adding resistance.

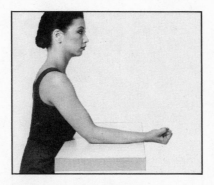

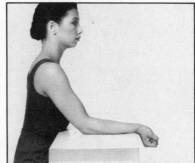

Level 5:

With your elbows either bent or straight, hold a bar with both hands, palms facing down. Alternating hands, roll the bar away from you.

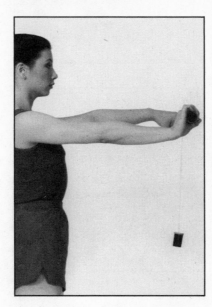

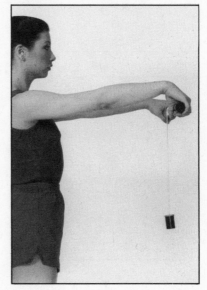

Wrist Radial Deviation

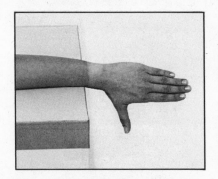 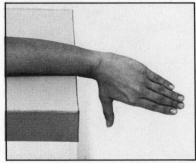

Level 1:
Sit with your forearm supported and thumb toward the floor. Bend your wrist down.

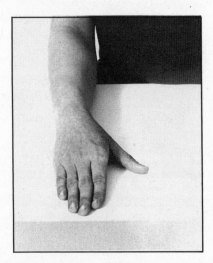 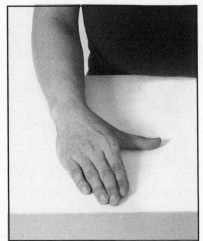

Level 2:
Sit with your arm bent, forearm supported and palm facing down. Bend your wrist inward toward the thumb.

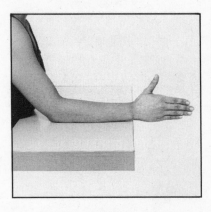 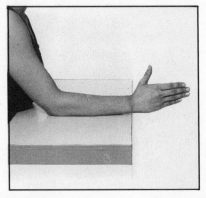

Level 3:
Sit or stand with your forearm supported, wrist straight, and thumb toward the ceiling. Bend your wrist up.

Level 4:
Same as level 3, adding resistance.

Level 5:

Stand with your arms straight out. With palms facing each other, hold a heavy stick or hammer pointing forward. Raise tip of resistance toward the ceiling.

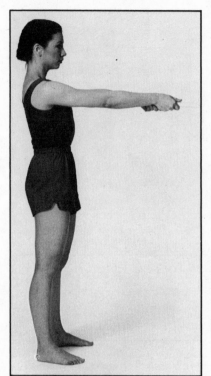 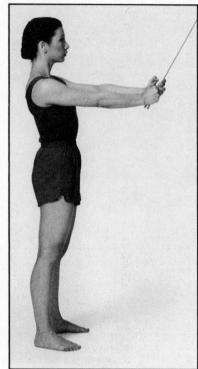

Wrist Ulnar Deviation

Level 1:

Sit with your forearm supported, thumb toward the ceiling. Bend your wrist down.

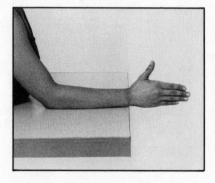 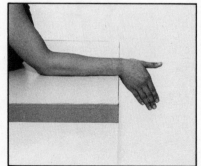

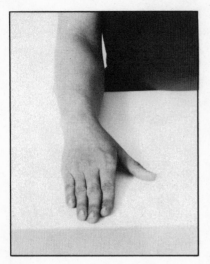 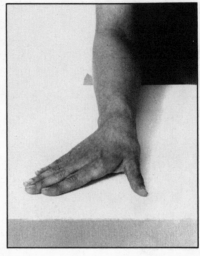

Level 2:
   Sit with your arm bent, forearm supported and palm facing down. Bend your wrist out toward the pinky finger.

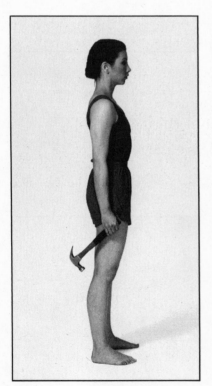 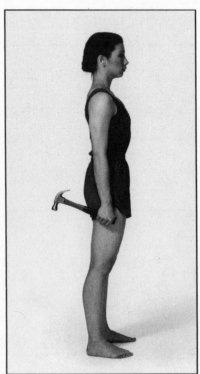

Level 3:
   Stand with your arm at your side and wrist in neutral position. Move your wrist back toward your pinky finger. (Refer to photo for level 4, without hammer.)

Level 4:
   Same as level 3, adding resistance.

Level 5:

Lie on your back with arms out straight. Hold an object of resistance, such as a pole, and move it so that it points toward the ceiling.

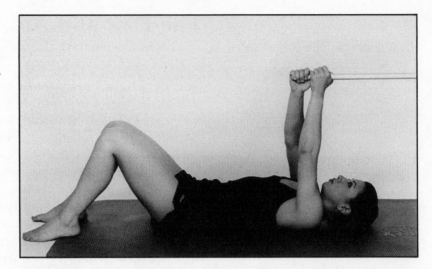

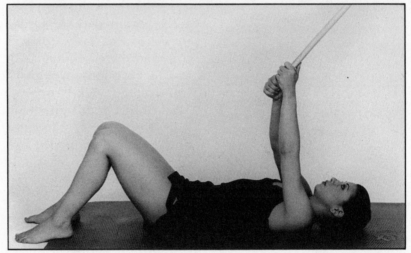

The Foot and Ankle

Oddly enough, I see as many ankle and foot injuries in non-athletes as I do in athletes. A great deal of wear and tear is placed on the ankles and feet as a result of the upright position alone. People who jog a couple of miles each day (not to mention those who run up to one hundred miles a week) place an even greater demand on this area of the body. Although runners sustain injuries from the repetitive banging of their feet and ankles against the pavement (or track), the stress is just as great for someone who climbs stairs, walks in high heels, or twists an ankle when stepping off a curb.

Perhaps the most common injury in all of sports is the sprained ankle. Usually one or both of the ligaments of the outer ankle is strained or torn. This is followed by swelling, pain, and, at times, muscle spasm. First and foremost: Ice it! Put ice on the ankle immediately, lightly massaging the area occasionally. Wait twenty-four hours before beginning a deep massage. Repeated sprains result in a stretching and loosening of the ligaments, causing greater instability in the area. Therefore, it is important that the area is made completely healthy as soon as possible with exercise and massage before resuming full activity on that leg.

The Achilles tendon is one of the body's thickest tendons. It connects the calf muscles with the heel bone and is responsible for allowing you to rise up on your toes, which is necessary for running and walking. Unless completely ruptured, where it would require surgery, the injury can be treated with my restorative methods.

Shinsplints are an occupational hazard to any runner. Muscle fibers on both sides of the shinbone swell and, in some cases, slightly tear from the extra stress.

Eamonn Coghlan had a severe case of shinsplints and stress fractures from the thousands of miles logged in his career. His ankle flexibility was poor, and the area was marked by unhealthy muscle tissue and the heavy formation of N-bodies. Since living regularly in the United States, Eamonn no longer was massaged regularly, and his ankles and shins were showing the signs of overuse by continually breaking down.

I applied two hours of tissue-restorative massage on Eammon's shins every night during the first stages of treatment. The soft tissue in the area became healthier, and Eamonn developed better flexibility and muscle condition, which allowed him to run more easily and successfully.

Jerry, who is in his late fifties, was experiencing terrible pain in the back of his foot from jogging. A specialist put him on a treadmill to analyze his gait and told him that his ankles were pronated and that there were loose bodies or bone chips in his ankle that had to be removed.

So Jerry had the surgery. Even after extended recuperation, no exercise therapy was prescribed for him, and his muscles atrophied from the inactivity, making the situation worse. Once he began running again, the pain returned. The problem, it was discovered, was actually an inflammation of the tendons along the inside of his Achilles. He needed twenty sessions of massage for that part of the foot to eliminate the pain, along with exercises to increase his strength.

Other injuries that are common to the foot and ankle are anterior tibialis tendonitis, a strained tendon along the inner arch of the foot; plantar fasciitis, a partial tear in the arch ligament on the bottom of the foot that is characterized by pain under the heel bone; extensor hallucis longus tendonitis, an injury running from the big toe diagonally across the foot to the ankle, which often plagues ballerinas who for long periods of time balance themselves on their toes or the balls of their feet; cruciate crural ligament sprain, which is felt along the top of the foot; interosseous strain, a tearing of the muscle that lies between the metatarsal bones of

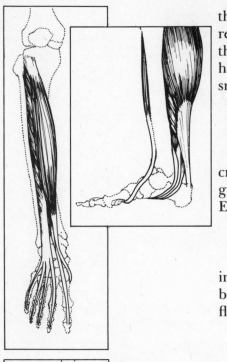

the foot and helps stabilize the front of the foot; and retrocalcaneal bursitis, an inflammation of the bursa that lies at the junction of the Achilles tendon and the heel bone and is the result of pressure from a shoe or sneaker.

Circle 1 - (front) Common injuries: shinsplints, cruciate crural ligament sprain, extensor hallucis longus tendonitis, extensor digitorum longus tendonitis. Exercise: ankle/foot flexion.

Circle 2 - (inside) Common injuries: shinsplints, inner ankle sprain, retinaculum injuries, posterior tibialis tendonitis. Exercises: ankle/foot inversion and flexion.

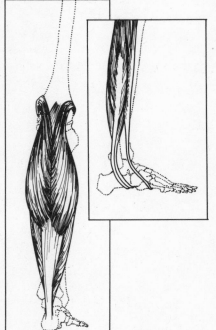

Circle 3 - (outside) Common injuries: outside ankle sprain, retinaculum injuries, peroneal tendonitis, shinsplints. Exercises: ankle/foot eversion and dorsiflexion.

Circle 4 - (back) Common injury: Achilles tendonitis. Exercise: ankle/foot plantar flexion and inversion.

Top of foot - Common injuries: Strains of the toe extensors, interosseous strain. Exercises: toe extension and ankle dorsiflexion.

Bottom of foot - Common injury: Plantar fasciitis. Exercise: Plantar flexion and dorsiflexion.

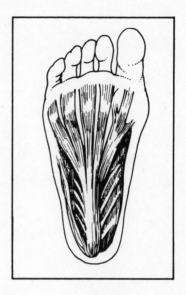

Massage

Top of Foot

1. Sit with your lower leg and foot supported in a comfortable position.

2. Spread cream over the top of the foot and shin.

3. Start with a superficial effleurage to the top of the foot and shin, using one or two hands.

4. Now do a deeper effleurage over the same area, working upward from the foot to the shin, using the heel of your hand or the first three fingers.

5. Continue with a deep effleurage, using the thumbs of both hands to massage each toe separately in deep, longitudinal strokes, including the soft tissue between the toes and massaging up the foot to the shin.

6. Now do a friction massage, using both thumbs

to make deep circles from the ankle up along either side of the shinbone.

7. Continue a friction massage, using the thumb to make deep circles outlining the anklebones.

8. Follow this with deep effleurage from the tips of the toes up along the top of the foot to the shin.

9. End with superficial effleurage from the tips of the toes up along the top of the foot to the shin.

Sole of the Foot

1. Lie on your stomach with your lower leg and foot supported on a pillow for comfort.

2. Follow the same massage steps as for the top of the foot. During the friction massage of steps 6 and 7, concentrate on massaging the arch.

Achilles Tendon

1. Lie on your stomach with your lower leg supported on a pillow for comfort.

2. Spread cream from the heel to the back of the knee.

3. Start with a superficial effleurage, using both hands from the heel to the back of the knee.

4. Now do a deeper effleurage to this same area, using the heels of both hands or the first three fingers of both hands.

5. Do petrissage now, using the thumb and first two fingers of both hands to knead the heel cord and calf.

6. Now begin a friction massage, using the thumbs of both hands to make deep circles along the sides of the heel cord and moving upward to the calf.

7. Repeat deep effleurage from the heel up to the shin.

8. End with a superficial effleurage along the same area.

Exercises

Special Exercises for Shinsplints

1. Stand with one leg resting from knee to foot on a bench. Sit on your foot.

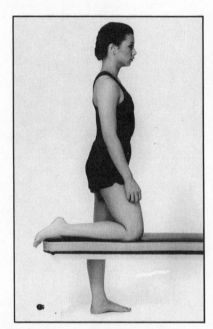 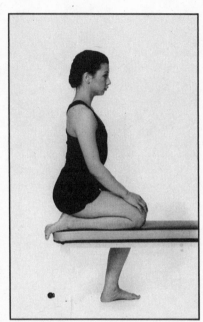

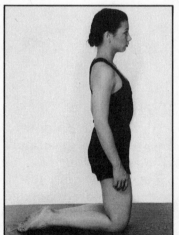 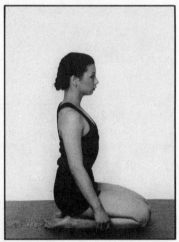 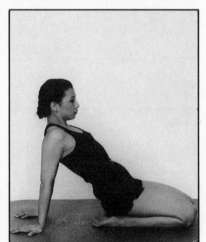

2. Kneel, then sit on both feet. Place both hands behind you on floor, moving them back until you are in a leaning position.

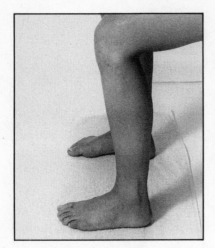 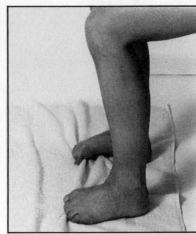

3. Sit on a chair or bench, with both feet resting on a towel on the floor. Curl your toes so that they grab the towel, then release.

Dorsiflexion

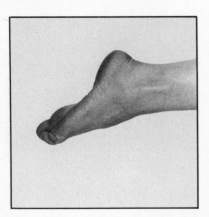 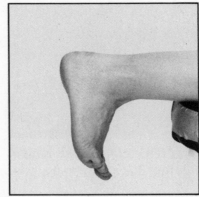

Level 1:

Lie stomach-down with your legs supported at the edge of a bench and your feet hanging over the edge. Move your toes toward your head.

Level 2:

Lie on your side and move your toes toward your head.

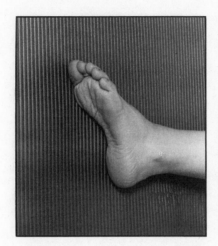 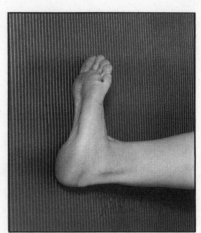

Level 3:

a. Sit on a chair with one or both feet dangling. Lift your toes toward your head, pointing them in, out, and also straight.

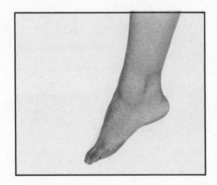 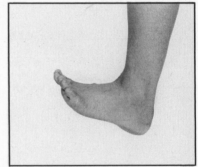

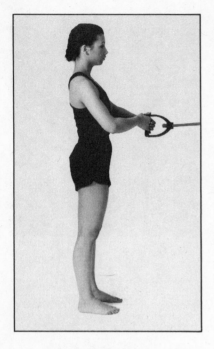

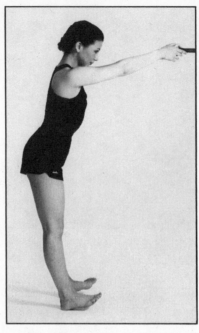

b. Holding a bar or cable for support, stand on your heels. Shift your weight back onto your heels.

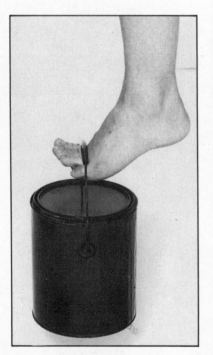

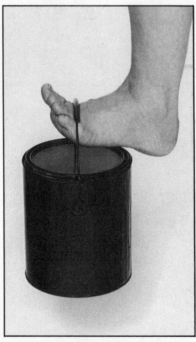

Level 4:
   Same as level 3a, adding resistance and lifting your toes only straight toward your head.

Level 5:
   Same as level 4, but also tilting your foot to the inside and outside while lifting up.

Plantar Flexion

Level 1:
Sit on the edge of a table. Begin with your toes pointing upward, then point your toes toward the floor.

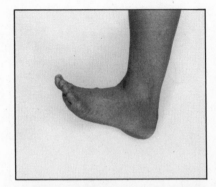 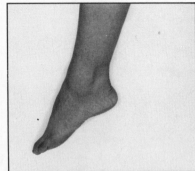

Level 2:
Lie on your side and point your toes downward.

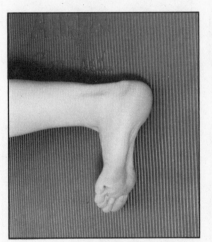 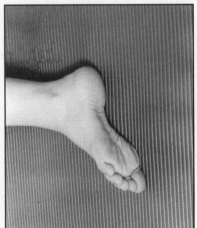

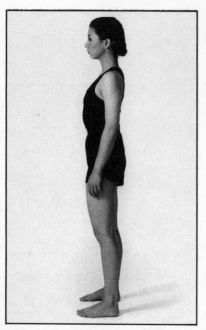

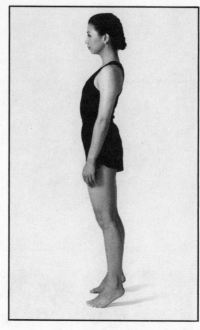

<u>*Level 3:*</u>
Sit or stand and lift your heels off the floor.

<u>*Level 4:*</u>
Same as level 3, adding resistance.

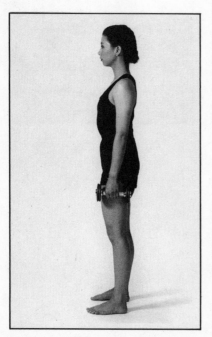

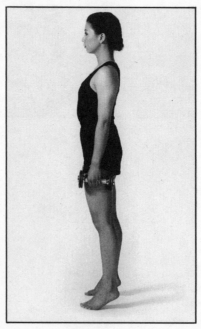

<u>*Level 5:*</u>
Same as level 4, placing the ball of your foot on the edge of a step or on top of a 2-inch board.

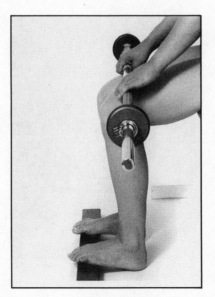
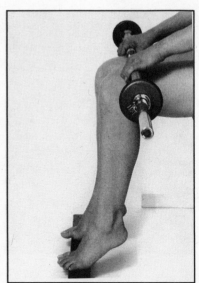

Foot Inversion

Level 1:
Lie on your side with your top leg resting on a bench. Move your foot down to the floor.

Level 2:
Lie on your back with your legs outstretched. Turn your foot inward.

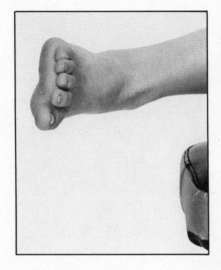
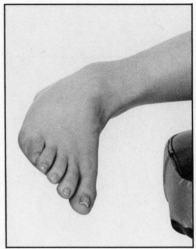

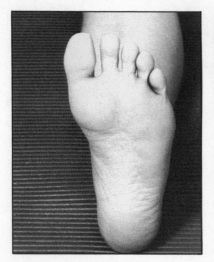

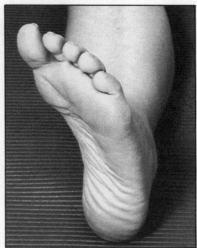

Level 3:

Lie on your side with your bottom leg supported at the ankle. Lift your foot toward the ceiling.

Level 4:

Same as level 3, adding resistance.

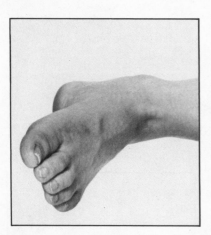

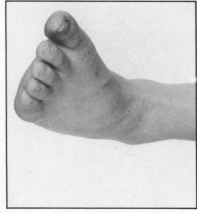

Level 5:

Sitting on the edge of a table and holding a can between both feet, bend your knees and bring them toward your chest.

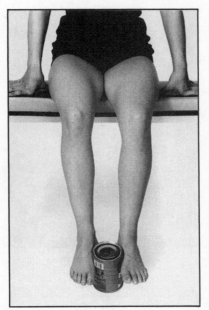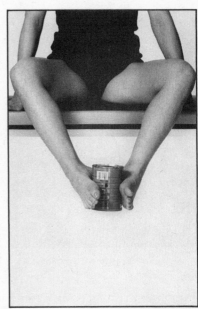

Foot Eversion

Level 1:

Lie on your side with your bottom leg supported at the ankle. Move your foot toward the floor.

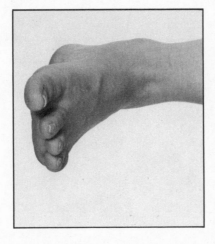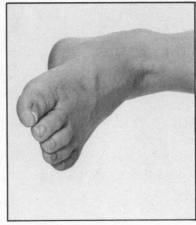

Level 2:

Lie on your back with your legs outstretched. Turn your foot outward.

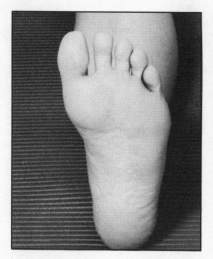 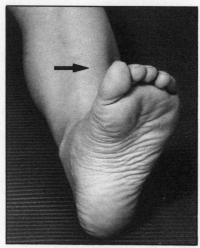

Level 3:

Lie on your side with your top leg supported at the ankle. Lift your foot toward the ceiling.

Level 4:

Same as level 3, adding resistance to the outside of your foot manually or with weights.

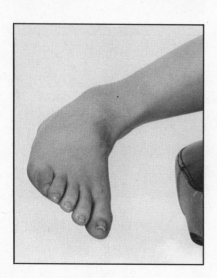 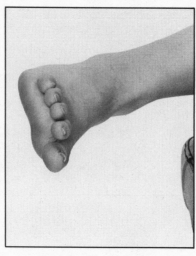

EPILOGUE

So, NOW YOU'RE ON YOUR OWN.

The Chasnov Method, through a program based on good posture and symmetry, restorative massage and exercise, has enabled you to heal your injuries, correct and prevent physical problems and improve your performance. An understanding and a belief in its philosophy, as well as a commitment to it in practice, should make your body better.

Yet, for some of you, the pain may linger, the problems may persist. What do you do if you're not getting the desired results?

If all of your personal efforts have failed, you should see a physical therapist for an evaluation. In most states, the law mandates that a person be referred to physical therapy by a physician. Some states, however, do not require a referral for an evaluation. A physician will refer a patient to physical therapy after X rays have determined that there are no broken bones, or a bone specialist has made that determination without X rays. Your best bet in choosing a physical therapist is to contact the American Physical Therapy Association (APTA) or its regional representative. These organizations can usually recommend a good physical therapist in your area. A last resort is to consult the telephone book.

You should also be aware of what a physical therapist can offer you. There are a number of different modalities they provide that can help relieve pain and return function in soft-tissue injuries, when combined with massage and exercise. By themselves, the heat, sound, electricity, and light treatments available are short-term solutions that may increase blood flow and break up muscle spasms, but alone will not get your body any healthier. Only massage and exercise can do that; everything else is simply a bonus.

Although several heat treatments can be done at home—for example, heat from hot packs, hot towels, or gauze—most of the advanced equipment is only found in a physical therapist's office. This equipment includes the following:

● MENS—microelectrical nerve stimulation. The Myomatic I uses minimal-intensity microstimulation as a form of electrotherapy to electrochemically reduce inflammation and stimulate the body's natural healing mechanism.

● Electrical stimulation—currents of electricity force the muscles to contract and relax, breaking the spasm and increasing the blood supply.

● Ultrasound—a form of microwave with high-frequency sound waves that decreases pain and increases blood circulation.

● Iontophoresis—electricity drives chemicals into the body to heal the injury.

● Interferential—two currents of lower intensity provide deeper relief for pain.

● Transcutaneous nerve stimulation—low level electrical currents are used to reduce pain.

● Cervical traction—manual and machine techniques gently separate the vertebrae in the neck or lower back to reduce pressure on the nerves.

● Mobilization—special manual joint movement techniques allow for greater mobility.

● Infrared/microwave diathermy—forms of heat from machines stimulate healing without ever coming in contact with the body.

● Manipulation—manual treatment of soft-tissue injuries other than by massage.

● Hot wax (or paraffin)—used primarily for fingers or toes to increase circulation to the area.

If you are unable to find someone to massage you, whether it be a relative, friend, or physical therapist, I recommend contacting a licensed massage therapist.

This book was written to provide you with a source, a self-help guide to making your body better. Even though you may not know exactly what is wrong with you or why or how it happened, you now have the ammunition to fight back. You've got in your corner the "technology" to take care of yourself. Chances are very good that you should be feeling better already. Good health!

INDEX

neck rotation, 105–6
healing, case examples, 98–100
massage of, 101
shock absorbers to, 98
support of, 98

Nervous system
    control of body, order of, 19
    effects of massage, 49
    signals to muscles, 18, 45

Neutral warmth, treating injuries, 85

O

One-repetition maximum (1 RM)
    method, 75

P

Pain
        referred pain, 94–95
        tolerance for, 44

Pelvis, 16

Petrissage, 55, 60

Physical therapy
    finding therapist, 195
    physical referral, 195
    treatments used by, 196

Plantar fasciitis, 181

Posture, 21–34
        changes over time, 22–23
        defintion of, 21–22
        developmental view, 27

effect on bodily systems, 23–24, 26
evolutionary view, 27
improvement of
    massage, 25–26
    stretching exercises, 28–34
    visualization, 28
poor posture, 23–25
    of athletes, 24–25, 35
    characteristics of, 23
    compensation of body, 24, 25
    muscle imbalances caused by,
        120–21

Power building phase, exercise
    program, 77

Progressive-resistance exercise, 69

Q

Quadriceps, 132

R

Rectus femoris, 132

Referred pain, 94–95

Rehabilitation phase, exercise program,
    77

Relative Repetition Maximum (RRM)
    method, evaluating functional level,
    75–76, 77

Repetitions, definition of, 73

Resistance exercises
    levels of difficulty, 93–94

About the Author

Marc Chasnov, M.A., R.P.T., is a licensed physical therapist with a graduate certificate from New York University and a Masters Degree in Movement Science from Teacher's College at Columbia University. He runs a thriving physical therapy clinic in Rye Brook, New York, specializing in the manual evaluation and treatment of soft tissue injuries by tissue restorative massage, and the prescription of therapeutic exercise. In addition, Marc is a member of the National Strength and Conditioning Association and the Science Advisory Board of Runner's World Magazine and coaches weight lifting. His female pupils have been finalists in state, national and World Championship Women's Olympic Weightlifting. He and his wife, Lorraine, make their home in Westchester County, New York.